90 0694376 7

Recent Research in

D1420284

Margaret A. Cormack R. Glynn Owens
Michael E. Dewey

Reducing Benzodiazepine Consumption

Psychological Contributions to
General Practice

Springer-Verlag
New York Berlin Heidelberg
London Paris Tokyo Hong Kong

Dr. Margaret A. Cormack
Department of Psychology
Washington Singer Laboratories
University of Exeter
Exeter EX4 4QG
England

Dr. R. Glynn Owens
Sub-Department of Clinical Psychology
Department of Psychiatry
New Medical School
University of Liverpool
Liverpool L69 3BX
England

Michael E. Dewey
Department of Psychiatry
Royal Liverpool Hospital
University of Liverpool
Liverpool L69 3BX
England

Library of Congress Cataloging-in-Publication Data
Cormack, Margaret A.
    Reducing benzodiazepine consumption : psychological contributions
to general practice / Margaret A. Cormack, R. Glynn Owens, Michael
E. Dewey.
        p.   cm.—(Recent research in psychology)
    Bibliography: p.
    ISBN 0-387-97035-5 (alk. paper)
    1. Benzodiazepines.   2. Drugs—Dosage—Reduction.   3. Medication
abuse—Prevention.   4. Chemotherapy—Psychological aspects.
    I. Owens, R. Glynn.   II. Dewey, Michael E.   III. Title.   IV. Series.
    RM666.B42C67   1989
    615'.7882—dc20   89-1150

Printed on acid-free paper

Camera-ready text provided by the authors.
Printed and bound by Edwards Brothers, Ann Arbor, Michigan.
Printed in the United States of America.

9 8 7 6 5 4 3 2 1

ISBN 0-387-97035-5 Springer-Verlag New York Berlin Heidelberg
ISBN 3-540-97035-5 Springer-Verlag Berlin Heidelberg New York

THE AUTHORS

Margaret A. Cormack, Lecturer in Clinical Psychology at the University of Exeter, conducted this work for her Ph.D. She has been involved in joint work with general practitioners in Mersey Region, North West Region, and South West Region for some years, providing research and educational resources.

R. Glynn Owens, now Senior Lecturer in Clinical Psychology in the Department of Psychiatry at the University of Liverpool, supervised this work. At the University of Liverpool he is involved in the training of clinical psychologists, doctors, and nurses, and at the same time conducts research in a number of areas relating to psychology and health. Recently, he was Lecturer in Research Methods in the Department of Psychology at the University College of North Wales In Bangor.

Michael E. Dewey, Lecturer in Psychological Statistics at the University of Liverpool, guided the research design and data analysis. With collaboration from psychiatry and clinical psychology, he works on the application of statistical and computing techniques to psychological research.

ACKNOWLEDGMENTS

For three years, this study was funded by Mersey Regional Health Authority, which contributed to the costs of conducting the research. Thanks are expressed to them for their generous help.

The doctors and receptionists in the practices gave freely of their time and energy to enable the project to run smoothly. Their efforts to assist in gaining information about the subjects were invaluable, and their friendliness and help made the work a pleasure.

Many thanks are given to Margaret Donnelly and Sandy Salisbury, who painstakingly typed the manuscript, and to Rachel Kirby, who unravelled the word processing knots.

CONTENTS

Part One: *Background to the Study*

Part Two: A Study of Drug Reduction

Outline of the Study

Results

Discussion

Comments on the Work

PART ONE: BACKGROUND TO THE STUDY

Introduction

In 1980 the first reports of dependence on therapeutic doses of benzodiazepines began to have an impact and the Committee on the Review of Medicines published a report detailing the ineffectiveness of long-term use of these drugs. General practitioners were faced with the possibility that they had many patients who not only were not benefitting from their medication, but who also might be dependent on the drugs and therefore might find it very difficult to stop taking benzodiazepines. The author (MC) and a local general practitioner discussed psychological approaches which might be useful in helping patients to reduce medication, and a project was devised to test the efficacy of anxiety management techniques as an alternative to benzodiazepine use.

The doctors in the practice wrote to the selected patients asking them to try to reduce their medication and inviting them to come to an interview with the psychologist to receive advice on how to cope without tablets. For those patients who came to interview, group work on anxiety management was offered and this proved to be moderately successful. However, the most interesting and unexpected finding was that those who did not attend the interview or take part in the group therapy similarly reduced their medication (Cormack & Sinnott, 1983). Over one-third of patients could reduce their drug-taking significantly, merely by receiving a letter from their doctor asking them to do so.

The results of the study were presented at the Merseyside and North Wales Faculty of the Royal College of General Practitioners. Interest in the findings led to a further project which forms the basis of this book. General practitioners who were involved in the teaching of undergraduate medical students and the training of general practitioners were selected from those who volunteered to take part in the research and a more detailed study of responses to doctors' requests to stop benzodiazepine medication was undertaken.

In the early 1980's clinical psychology was starting to move into the community and, following the Trethowan Report (1977), closer links with primary care were established. Not only did this project fit with the directives of the report to increase research activity, but it also led to a number of educational activities. Michael Forrest, then a course organiser in the vocational training for general practitioners, and Margaret Cormack set up a number of workshops on benzodiazepine prescribing which attracted GPs and other primary health care workers.

Also, at the time of the project, general practitioner trainers were invited to a recurrent series of workshops on teaching consultation skills. The author (MC) and other psychologists contributed in teaching psychological aspects of interviewing. In many ways this work could be viewed as central to the issue of preventing long term use of benzodiazepines. If doctors gain confidence and skills in interviewing, then they may feel that they are providing a better service for patients by listening and counselling, and thus may not need to sign a prescription for benzodiazepines so often.

Many of the problems that people bring to the general practitioner are not medical and thus are not appropriately resolved by drugs. It is the case that many people could benefit from referral to clinical psychology services, but in Britain there are far too few clinical psychologists for all patients to be offered this service (approximately 1,700 clinical psychologists were in NHS posts in 1987). The ways in which clinical psychologists and GPs will best work together in the future may be in projects of the kind described in this book and in increased collaboration in continuing education.

Literature Review

1. INTRODUCTION

The literature to be discussed covers a number of aspects of the use of
benzodiazepines. Although benzodiazepines have been very widely
prescribed, the therapeutic effectiveness of the drugs may be questioned,
both in short-term use and in longer-term therapy which is often
administered through repeat prescriptions. Effects of the drugs on
psychomotor and cognitive performance indicate deficits which can affect
normal day to day functioning.

An important feature in understanding the long-term use of benzodiazepines
is an identification of reasons for prescribing and use in different
socio-demographic groups. Whether the benzodiazepines produce classical
dependence in long-term users is a moot point. If benzodiazepines are to
be used less, then it may be conjectured that alternatives may be
psychological methods of dealing with life's difficulties.

2. THE BENZODIAZEPINES

2.1 History of the benzodiazepines

In comparison with the barbiturates, the benzodiazepines performed a
similar function, acting as hypnotics, but were safe in overdose, and for
this reason alone were viewed as preferable. At the time they were first
developed and marketed, they were thought to be non-addictive (Owen and
Tyrer, 1983; Edwards et al, 1984), another advantage over the
barbiturates, and they soon replaced the older drugs as the medication of
choice for insomnia and anxiety. The first three drugs were introduced by
Hoffman la Roche: Librium in 1960, followed by Valium and Mogadon. Until
the restricted list in 1985, when only a few benzodiazepines were
available by their generic names on National Health Service prescriptions,
these drugs were very commonly prescribed and they have become household
names. Table 1 lists the most popular benzodiazepines with their year of
introduction.

TABLE 1

Year of clinical introduction of commonly prescribed benzodiazepines

Year	Drug
1960	Chlordiazepoxide (Librium)
1962	Diazepam (Valium)
1965	Nitrazepam (Mogadon)
	Oxazepam (Serenid-D)
1970	Flurazepam (Dalmane)
1972	Clorazepate (Tranxene)
1975	Lorazepam (Ativan)

Source: Allgulander (1978).

2.2 Pharmacological action of the benzodiazepines

Benzodiazepine receptors in the brain facilitate the action of GABA-ergic systems, GABA (gamma-amino-butyric acid) being a widespread inhibitory neurotransmitter (Gray, 1979; Lader, 1979). Benzodiazepine receptors have been found scattered over large areas of the brain with heavy concentrations in the neocortex and septo-hippocampal system. The clinical anti-anxiety action may be due to limbic system depression (Greenblatt and Shader, 1974) and the septo-hippocampal system may play a central role in mediating anxiety (Gray, 1979).

Both the benzodiazepines and the barbiturates enhance the effects of GABA: the benzodiazepines may act presynaptically to increase the amount of GABA released or to increase the sensitivity of the GABA-ergic interneurons to excitatory influences. Alternatively, the action may be postsynaptically to increase the efficacy of GABA at the synaptic membrane.

So far, an endogenous ligand for benzodiazepine receptors has not been found, although Hollister (1981) hypothesised that high trait anxiety could be the result of deficiencies in the ligand. This might suggest that people with high trait anxiety would be more likely to become dependent on benzodiazepines.

2.3 Different types of benzodiazepines

All benzodiazepines can act as hypnotics or tranquillisers according to dosage, although those with a short duration of action (such as temazepam) are at present more popular as hypnotics because they do not produce a hangover effect in the morning (Hindmarch 1979a). Most of the benzodiazepines have active metabolites and thus the therapeutic effect of the drug may continue for some time. All of the benzodiazepines to a greater or lesser extent share the following actions: anti-anxiety, sedative/ hypnotic, muscle relaxant, anti-convulsant and amnestic.

Lorazepam was developed as a drug without active metabolites, with the aim of being useful for the necessary period of time and no longer, and therefore being appropriate for panic attacks or conditions where anxiety was intermittent. However, it now appears that the rapid onset and cessation of the anti-anxiety effect of the drug may be contributing to the development of dependence through a severe withdrawal reaction (Tyrer et al, 1981; Hollister, 1981; Petursson and Lader, 1984).

In terms of pharmacological structure, all of the available benzodiazepines in Britain except one are 1,4 benzodiazepines. The exception is clobazam, a 1,5 benzodiazepine, which has less sedative and muscle relaxant effects and produces less psychomotor impairment following administration of single or repeated doses (Hindmarch, 1979b; Hindmarch and Parrott, 1979). Throughout the book, except where specified, the term "benzodiazepine" will refer to compounds in the 1,4 class of benzodiazepines. The differences between the drugs are often described in terms of half-life variations, but this may not be a useful guide to the differences in effects of the drugs for a number of reasons. (Examples of half-lives of commonly prescribed benzodiazepines are shown in Table 2.)

Garattini et al (1979) demonstrated dramatic inter-individual differences in half-lives of benzodiazepines. Subjects were given a single oral dose of 15 mg of diazepam and three hours later the measured blood levels of the drug differed between subjects by a factor of 20. Plasma half-lives of the drugs may be prolonged in the elderly through decreased clearance or increased volume of distribution (Mendelson,1980), so a dosage that may be recommended for a young adult may be toxic for the elderly.

Hindmarch (1985) has stressed that the nature and duration of a drug's clinical activity are not necessarily related to the drug's half-life, but depend on the rate of absorption, the time to peak plasma concentration, the shape of the pharmacokinetic curve and the plasma concentration corresponding to the threshold for clinical activity. Drugs with a long half-life will accumulate to a steady state achieved after an interval of four times the half-life (Greenblatt et al, 1981).

TABLE 2

Half-lives of benzodiazepines and active metabolites in healthy adults

Drug	Half-life of the Parent Drug (Hours)	Half-life of the Active Metabolites (Hours)
Nitrazepam (Mogadon)	18 - 30*	-
Flurazepam (Dalmane)	very short	24 - 28
Diazepam (Valium)	14 - 90	31, 8, 30-60, 4 -10
Temazepam (Normison/ Euhypnos)	4 - 10	-
Oxazepam (Serenid-D)	6 - 24	-
Triazolam (Halcion)	5 - 10	3 - 10
Chlordiazepoxide (Librium)	7 - 14	
Lorazepam (Ativan)	9 - 22	-
Clorazepate (Tranxene)	-	30 - 60

Source: Breimer, 1979
* Breimer et al, 1977.

In recent years, there has been a trend towards producing hypnotics with a short half-life to avoid the problem of hangover effect in the morning. Unfortunately, these are not without drawbacks: daytime anxiety has been shown to increase after taking triazolam at night (Morgan & Oswald, 1982; Oswald,1983). Triazolam is eliminated within four hours after ingestion and it has been postulated that it is the very rapid change in drug levels which provokes the day-time anxiety.

6

2.4 The therapeutic effect of the benzodiazepines

There is controversy over how useful the drugs are for anxiety and insomnia and some distinctions have been made which might identify populations likely or not to respond to benzodiazepine medication.

a) Use as anxiolytics

A number of authors have highlighted the lack of effectiveness of the benzodiazepines: Lader (1981a) described the long-term use of benzodiazepines as an expensive waste of effort; Harris et al (1977) demonstrated that psychoactive drugs had no curative effect in terms of psychoneurotic status; Salkind et al (1979) found a high placebo response to vitamin C in comparison with clobazam 10 and diazepam 5; Catalan and Gath (1985) reported that benzodiazepines were not effective with patients with low levels of anxiety; and Hollister (1973), in reviewing the use of anti-anxiety drugs in clinical practice, found that drugs were not distinguished from placebo in patients with chronic anxiety reinforced by social, interpersonal or economic problems.

Patients who may benefit from treatment with benzodiazepines have been identified: Rickels (1973) found that high somatization of complaints predicted improvement with diazepam rather than with chlordiazepoxide or placebo. This was explained in terms of the muscle relaxant properties of diazepam. However, irrespective of treatment, patients with higher education, higher income and a realisation that their problems were emotional improved more than others. This implies that personal resources play an important role in the success of treatment.

By 1980, Rickels had qualified the class of responders to benzodiazepines as non-psychotic anxious patients, suffering primarily from emotional and somatic symptoms of anxiety rather than from depression and interpersonal problems. In 1983, Rickels reported that at one year follow-up, 60% of those who were treated successfully with diazepam for six weeks to six months had become symptomatic again. This was interpreted as evidence that treatment of several months or years duration is appropriate for a significant sub-group of chronically anxious patients. However, an alternative explanation could be that the drugs suppressed any other strategies that could have been employed to cope with or eliminate the anxiety, and that long-term drug use was thus inappropriate for these individuals.

Catalan and Gath (1985) reported that benzodiazepines undermined the individual's capacity to draw on personal resources to cope with adversity. They suggested that benzodiazepines should be used only for severe anxiety and then only for a period of up to three weeks with concurrent work to investigate the causes of the anxiety. In a similar vein, Higgitt et al (1985) indicated that benzodiazepines should not be prescribed for normal people at times of acute stress such as a divorce or bereavement, and they suggested that brief counselling could be effective for minor psychological disorders. The role of the doctor in patient expectations has been highlighted by Helman (1981) who argued that doctors communicate a model for dealing with problems which does not allow the patient to confront the problem but suppresses anxiety with the aid of a pharmacological prop. Parish (1982) expounded that the demand for medical intervention has been created by doctors through a widescale medicalization of life's trials and tribulations. Thus there is a need for doctors to become more skilled in counselling techniques to help patients to find their own solutions to problems.

b) Use as hypnotics

Although benzodiazepines have been shown to aid sleep, the effectiveness of the drugs can be minimal within a few weeks, or daytime anxiety can be produced by them. Oswald's work in sleep-laboratory studies showed that poor sleepers fell asleep more quickly and slept on average 50 minutes longer after nitrazepam (Adam and Oswald, 1982). By the third week, however, there was no shortening of sleep latency; and sleep duration, although longer than at baseline, was shorter than in the first week of ingestion. Tedeschi et al (1985) also demonstrated tolerance to the sedative action of nitrazepam after six nights, but found no tolerance to temazepam, a shorter-acting drug.

Differences in effectiveness of hypnotics are related to the half-life of the drug. With long-acting compounds, hypnotic efficacy peaks after some consecutive nights of drug taking (Kales, 1980; Roth et al, 1981). Changes in quality of sleep have been noted with nitrazepam, with small decreases in rapid eye movement sleep (REM) in the early part of the night and a reduction by half of slow wave sleep (stages 3 and 4) by the third week (Oswald, 1983). Kales & Scharf (1973) found that there was no stage 4 sleep in chronic users of diazepam. They reported that clinical doses of benzodiazepines did not produce a decrease in REM sleep but that higher doses did reduce REM sleep. However, Nicholson (1979a) suggested that hypnotics may often delay the onset of REM sleep and thus may lead to an overall reduction in amount of REM sleep.

Marks and Nicholson (1984) advised limited prescribing of the benzodiazepines for insomnia. They suggested that a rapidly eliminated hypnotic would be advisable with transient insomnia only if other approaches such as environmental change were ineffective. With short term insomnia related to an emotional or medical problem, three weeks maximum use of hypnotics was recommended, and intermittent use within this period would be desirable. For chronic insomnia, use for one night in three for up to a month was recommended. If this proved ineffective, then anti-depressant medication should be tried.

c) Benzodiazepines as therapy for depression

The benzodiazepines are not infrequently prescribed for depression, either alone or with an anti-depressant (Johnson, 1983). Women are more likely than men to be given benzodiazepines for depression (Clare and Williams, 1981) although the authors speculated that women may be more likely to present with depression in combination with anxiety. The boundary between anxiety and depression is not clear-cut and there is a correlation between anxiety symptoms and the core symptoms of depression (Cassano and Conti, 1981). Johnstone et al (1980) suggested that the distinction between anxiety and depression was of no practical value with regard to drug treatment, finding that amitryptiline improved both anxiety and depression, whereas diazepam was less effective with both.

d) Use of the benzodiazepines in physical illness

Mellinger and Balter's (1981) USA survey indicated that new therapy with an anti-anxiety agent was at least as likely for patients with a primary diagnosis of physical disorder as for those with a diagnosis of mental disorder. Cummins et al (1982) in a survey of over 7,000 middle-aged men found a strong positive link between tranquilliser use and the presence of a doctor-diagnosed physical disease mostly ischaemic heart disease and hypertension. A variety of physical diagnoses have led to prescriptions for minor tranquillisers: cardiovascular disease, insomnia secondary to pain due to musculoskeletal disorders, gastrointestinal disorders, respiratory disease, neoplasms and, in particular, rheumatic diseases

9

(Williams, 1978). Williams cited a study by Knight (1970) who had found that within a hospital setting the major source of out-patient prescriptions for diazepam was the department of physical medicine and rheumatology. The benzodiazepines have muscle relaxant effects and thus are useful to help relieve pain and control muscular spasm.

In a prospective study of 153 GP patients, Williams et al (1982) reported that 16% of the sample received psychotropic drugs for physical complaints within the six month study period. For hospital patients, the figures were even higher. Greenblatt and Shader (1974) reported an American study which found that in 1973, of all medical patients hospitalised in the Boston area, 32% received diazepam. To some extent, the use of benzodiazepines in hospital is for patient management (eg, the widespread use of hypnotics at night, whether necessary or not) rather than for treatment of features of the patient's illness.

    e) Paradoxical drug reactions

Although the benzodiazepines are known as tranquillisers, some reports have indicated that their effects are far from producing tranquillity in the individual. Hall and Zisook (1981), in discussing paradoxical reactions to benzodiazepines, suggested that the sedative effects of tranquillising drugs often interfere with other activities of the individual which serve as defences against conflict. The result of the blocking of these activities may be depression or hostility. Hall and Joffe (1972) reported a study which had been prompted by two patients who showed adverse effects to less than 40 mg of diazepam per day for six and eight days respectively. They monitored out-patients and found ten patients who demonstrated a number of symptoms which had appeared since starting diazepam therapy less than 30 days previously. The new symptoms included tremulousness, apprehension, confusion, insomnia, depression and ego-alien suicidal ideation (ie, feeling like killing themselves but not really wanting to die). The symptoms resolved within seven days of discontinuation of medication. Six patients were followed up for one year and no recurrence of symptoms was reported.

Greenblatt and Shader (1974) commented that minor tranquillisers could produce an apparently paradoxical increase in aggression if fear or anxiety were serving to inhibit aggression or hostility. In animal studies that they cited, attack aggression was resistant to chlordiazepoxide and they concluded that the animals experienced disinhibition and thus were able to express behaviour which previously would have been suppressed by punishment (see also Haefely, 1980). In humans, Greenblatt and Shader reported work by Feldman (1962) indicating a progressive development of .dislikes or hates in patients receiving diazepam.

Although a benzodiazepine may be given with the intention of helping a patient to deal better with stress, it may have the opposite effect. Gray et al (1983) suggested that benzodiazepines can impair the normal development of stress tolerance, through affecting a behavioural inhibition system whose function is to respond to warnings of punishment. Anecdotal evidence has linked the taking of tranquillisers by parents with actual or threatened child abuse (Lynch et al, 1975). There may be many factors leading to child abuse, and the taking of tranquillisers may be a response to these factors rather than contributing to the abuse in its own right. However, the role of benzodiazepines in impairing stress tolerance and releasing aggression in animals would indicate that the drugs may well be implicated in human violence.

2.5 Effects of benzodiazepines on performance

The studies on the effects of the drugs on performance must be viewed according to the subjects used. If the drugs work to reduce arousal, then, according to the Yerkes Dodson curve, performance of an anxious patient may be better after administration of an anxiolytic, but that of a non-anxious subject would be worse. The common side effect of sedation may wear off after several days and thus the performance of a long-term user may be different from that of a novice.

a) Effects in normal and anxious subjects

Lader et al (1980) followed healthy volunteer subjects over 14 days of a single daily dose and found that clorazepate dipotassium increased EEG fast-wave activity, produced some psychomotor impairments and resulted in subjective reports of a lowering of alertness. After 15 days, the psychomotor performance decrements were minimal, but performance on a digit symbol substitution task had deteriorated and the subjective ratings of alertness had decreased. Other work (Petursson & Lader, 1981) reported that improvement on the digit symbol substitution test occurred after withdrawal of benzodiazepines, indicating a direct effect of benzodiazepines on performance involving speed of movement and matching.

Nicholson & Spencer (1982) disputed the conclusions from the study, arguing that scores on the task improved over time in normal subjects and, thus, that the results showed the effects of learning rather than a drug effect. However, this argument does not explain the deterioration in performance on the digit symbol substitution task while taking the drug, and, thus, the evidence would point to a direct effect of the drug on performance, reversible once the drug is discontinued.

Hindmarch (1979) argued that the pathologically anxious or insomniac patient may be a better performer following treatment with benzodiazepines, but that many non-pathological individuals are receiving these drugs and suffering performance decrements. In particular, driving may be impaired because the sedative activity of 1,4 benzodiazepines can severely impair the regulation and performance of sensory motor tasks. Skegg et al (1979) demonstrated a highly significant association between the use of minor tranquillisers and the risk of serious road accident to drivers in a study of 43,117 subjects, linking GP prescriptions to records of hospital admissions and deaths. In a comparative study, Hindmarch (1981) showed that general car driving ability was impaired with lorazepam but not with clobazam, a benzodiazepine with less sedative effect than others.

A number of studies have detailed the performance impairments produced by the benzodiazepines. Linnoila (1983) summarized the major effects of various benzodiazepines, showing that the lowering of arousal can lead to unsteadiness, slowing of motor performance, impairment in information processing, and deficits in manual dexterity, tracking, vigilance and cognitive performance. It was found that clobazam raised arousal. It is interesting to note that severely anxious outpatients were impaired to the same degree after diazepam as were healthy volunteers.

In reviewing the literature on performance impairments produced by benzodiazepines, Lader (1983a) listed the most sensitive tests which discriminate between a benzodiazepine and placebo as: learning and memory tasks, tests involving speed and matching skills, and measures of general arousal.

Insensitive tests are those involving complex visual motor coordination, visual spatial performance and auditory perception. Thus it is the well established higher mental faculties which are least affected and learning, memory and simple repetitive tasks which are most affected (Wittenborn, 1979).

12

b) Decrements produced by hypnotics

Nicholson's substantial work on the effects on performance of benzodiazepines demonstrated that diazepam and temazepam reduced sleep onset latencies and increased total sleep time, but also reduced awake activity in young adults. In middle-aged patients, sleep was not improved, but they did suffer the side effect of day-time activity being reduced (Nicholson, 1981). Generally, when hypnotics are taken, performance can be impaired the next morning. Nitrazepam (10 mg), flurazepam (30 mg) and oxazepam (45 mg) are all likely to produce performance impairments the next morning, whereas clobazam does not lead to obvious decrements (Nicholson, 1979b). Performance on a card sorting task was shown to be impaired in normal (non-anxious) subjects 13 hours after taking nitrazepam and, by EEG measures, subjects were still drowsy 18 hours after the drug was taken (Malpas et al, 1970). A sobering report by Prescott (1983) showed from traffic accident statistics that benzodiazepines contributed significantly to traffic accidents, often in the morning after taking a hypnotic at night. A patient taking nitrazepam at night could have up to 85% of the dose in the body the following morning.

c) Cognitive impairments

Shader and Grenblatt (1981) reported a time-limited anterograde amnesia syndrome, similar to a Korsakoff syndrome, in some patients receiving lorazepam. The temporary nature of the deficit is called into question by the findings of Lader et al (1984) who compared brain scans of normals, alcoholics and long-term benzodiazepine users. The scans of the benzodiazepine users showed ventricular enlargement, indicating brain atrophy, although this was not as marked as in the alcoholic group.

Comparisons of patients at a pain treatment centre demonstrated the effects of benzodiazepines on cognitive performance (Hendler et al,1980). Patients were compared on a battery of psychometric tests, including intelligence test items, memory tasks and visuo-spatial tests. Those taking benzodiazepines, alone or in combination with narcotics, were significantly more impaired than those taking narcotics alone or those taking no medication. The study did not detail the length of time for which the drugs had been taken, but as all patients had chronic pain, it is probable that the drugs had been taken for some considerable period.

d) Effects in the elderly

Because of the differential effects of the benzodiazepines according to age, normal therapeutic doses can have toxic effects in the elderly.

Kaplan (1980) suggested that the increase in half-life of diazepam was as much as one hour per year of life. The effect of this is that the drug accumulates substantially in elderly patients. Even 5 mg of nitrazepam per night can be enough to produce a syndrome of disability with postural hypotension leading to falls, general deterioration, incontinence, inability to wake, confusion, dysarthria and disorientation (Evans and Jarvis, 1972). The effects are reversible on removal of the drug.

3. PRESCRIBING

3.1 Trends in prescribing

Mellinger and Balter (1981) found the numbers of prescriptions issued for psychotherapeutic drugs from drug stores in the USA increased by 75% between 1964 and 1973 and then decreased by 23% between 1973 and 1979. Rickels (1981) commented on a reduction from 104 million prescriptions for anxiolytics in 1973 to 87 million in 1978 by pointing out that the later prescriptions contained, in general, more tablets and tablets of larger size, so that actual consumption probably did not fall as much as might be assumed.

In England, Parish (1973) commented on an increase by nearly half in psychotropic drug prescribing between 1961 and 1971. This was partly due to sales promotion and partly due to the increasing number of people on long-term drug therapy. Mapes and Williams (1979) reported that between 1970 and 1975 the percentage increase in items of prescription was ten times as much as the percentage increase in the population in the same period, and the authors commented on a growing tendency to give a prescription when advice would be more useful. During the same period there was a reduction by half in the prescribing of barbiturate hypnotics and an increase of one third in non-barbiturate hypnotics (primarily

14

benzodiazepines), leading to an overall reduction in hypnotic prescribing of 12%. However, prescriptions for tranquillisers increased by 28% (Williams,1981). (Information was not given about the amount and dosage prescribed.)

3.2 Extent of use of the benzodiazepines

Various surveys have assessed the extent of use of psychotropic drugs (Literature summaries 1 and 2). The largest was that of Balter and colleagues which looked at national samples from nine Western European countries (Balter et al, 1974) and the USA (Mellinger and Balter, 1981). In the United Kingdom they found that 8.6% of the population had used anti-anxiety/sedative drugs daily for at least a month and that 14.2% had used the drugs at some time in the year prior to the survey. Other studies indicated fairly similar usage patterns, with figures for population use of all psychotropic drugs as 12.5% (King et al,1982), and 19% (Skegg et al, 1977). Figures for population use of sedatives and hypnotics were: 7.4% males and 15.8% females (Skegg et al, 1977), and for hypnotics, 3% females and 2.1% males (Mellinger and Balter, 1981).

In a survey of twelve GPs, eight per cent of consultations resulted in a prescription for hypnotics or sedatives (Berkeley and Richardson, 1973), and in a prospective study by Bass and Baskerville (1981) one third of patients with specific emotional complaints received minor tranquillisers within six months. Fleming and Cross (1984) reported that 20.6 prescriptions for psychotropic drugs were issued per 1,000 list size in general practice and Tyrer (1978) found that three quarters of patients referred by GPs to psychiatry were taking psychotropic drugs.

For the benzodiazepines alone, Skegg et al (1977) reported that diazepam was given to 6.1% of all people in the population and Lader (1983b) calculated that one in five women and one in ten men took the drugs during any one year, two thirds of these taking them for at least one month. The mean daily dose of diazepam was found to be 8.9 mg by King et al (1982), and the mean daily dose of nitrazepam was 7.5 mg.

Literature summary 1

Extent of use of the benzodiazepines and other psychotropic drugs

AUTHOR & PLACE	FIGURES OF USE
Balter et al, 1974 UK national survey	14.2% used anti-anxiety and sedative drugs during the previous year.
Mellinger and Balter, 1981. USA national survey	14.1% females and 7.5% males used a medically prescribed anti-anxiety agent in the year prior to interview. 3% females and 2.1% males used hypnotics in the previous year. 5.5% of the adult population used anti-anxiety drugs for less than one month in the year prior to interview.
King et al, 1982. Northern Ireland GP prescribing data.	12.5% of the adult population received psychotropic drugs in 1975 benzoidiazepines accounted for three-quarters of psychotropic drugs prescribed in 1980). Mean dose of diazepam = 8.9 mg/day. Mean dose of nitrazepam = 7.5 mg/day.
Lader 1983,b UK.	One in five women and one in ten men take benzodiazepines during any one year, two thirds of these for at least one month.
Skegg et al, 1977 UK	19% of people aged 15 and over received psychotropic drugs during one year. Sedatives were given to 7.4% males and 15.8% females during one year. Diazepam was given to 6.1% of all people in the population.
Berkeley and Richardson, 1973. UK. Survey of 7,379 consultations of 12 GPs.	Hypnotics and sedatives were prescribed in 8% of consultations tranquillisers in 6%.

Fleming and Cross, 1984
UK. Practice activity
analysis of 269 doctors.

20.6 prescriptions for psychotropic
drugs issued per 1,000 list size,
153 prescriptions for psychotropic
drugs per 1,000 consultations.

Tyrer, 1978
UK. Survey of patients
attending psychiatric out-
patients clinic.

3/4 of patients referred by GPs to
psychiatrists were taking
psychotropic drugs.

Bass and Baskerville
1981. Canada. Prospective
study of 223 family
practice patients.

One third of patients with specific
emotional complaints had received
minor tranquillisers within a six
month period.

Chronic use (ie daily for at least one year) of anti-anxiety agents was
estimated as occurring in 1.6% of the American population (Mellinger and
Balter, 1981). Lader (1983b) reported that 1.5% of the adult population
of Britain took benzodiazepines every day of the year. The UK survey of
Balter et al (1974) showed that 8.6% of the adult population reported
regular daily use for at least one month. In a survey of people
prescribed Valium, two thirds had used the drug for at least one year
(Tessler et al, 1978) and Tyrer (1978) found that 28% of psychiatric
out-patients who took psychotropic drugs had taken them for more than one
year.

Literature summary 2
Extent of chronic use of the benzodiazepines and other
psychotropic drugs

AUTHOR & PLACE	FIGURES OF USE
Balter et al, 1974 UK National survey.	8.6% of the adult population had regular daily use for at least one month of anti-anxiety/sedative drugs.
Mellinger and Balter, 1981. USA National survey.	1.6% demonstrated daily use of medically prescribed anti-anxiety agents over one year.
Lader, 1983b UK.	1.5% of the adult population took benzodiazepines every day of the year, and half of those had taken them for more than seven years.
Tessler et al, 1978 USA. Questionnaire to people prescribed Valium.	One in seven of people prescribed Valium used the drug for less than one month, two thirds used the drug for at least one year.
Tyrer, 1978 UK. Survey of patients attending psychiatric out-patient clinic.	28% of patients taking psychotropic drugs had taken them for more than one year.

3.3 Sex differences in the use of benzodiazepines

Evidence from a number of studies indicates that twice as many women as
men consume benzodiazepines (Literature summary 3). To explain this
finding, it could be hypothesized that women present more with complaints
likely to lead to a prescription of benzodiazepines, or, alternatively,
that the prescription is more likely to be given if the patient is female.
There is some support for both hypotheses.

Salkind (1981), in a quota sampling survey in Great Britain, found that
women score as more anxious than men on the Morbid Anxiety Inventory and
thus may be more likely to present with anxiety symptoms to the doctor.

Cooperstock (1971, 1978) argued that because women in Western society are allowed to express their feelings more than men are, they would be more likely to perceive emotional problems in themselves and thence to present to the doctor. Men, on the other hand, might be more likely to resort to self-medication, particularly in the form of alcohol, due to the greater ease of access to pubs. However, the actual difference in likelihood of presentation of symptoms is small, according to Ingham (1981), and would not account for the differences in consumption.

In more general terms, Dunnell (1973) showed that women reported more symptoms than men and were larger consumers of medicines at all ages. Shepherd's work (Shepherd et al, 1966) demonstrated that twice as many women as men are diagnosed as suffering from psychiatric illness and thus, presumably, are more likely to receive psychotropic medication. Whether this figure represents a true difference in incidence of psychiatric illness or results from the (predominantly male) medical view of women's presentation of emotional problems is a moot point.

There is some evidence to suggest that when patients go to the doctor, women are more likely than men to be prescribed benzodiazepines for the same presenting problems. Varnum (1981) reported that a higher proportion of men were not given psychotropic medication when they attended the GP with psychological problems. Similarly, Anderson (1981) reported that women aged between 25 and 44 years received prescriptions for anxiolytics significantly more often than men who had been given the same diagnosis. A prospective study by Williams et al (1982) found that men who complained of depression were likely to be prescribed anti-depressants, whereas a proportion of women with the same complaint were prescribed tranquillisers instead.

Literature summary 3
Sex differences in the use of benzodiazepines

Author	Male-female ratios	Comments
Cooperstock (1971,1978)	1:2	Women consume larger quantities than men.
Anderson (1981)	more women	For the same diagnosis women aged 25-44 received prescriptions for anxiolytics more often than men.
Balter et al (1974)	1:2	Women over 55 years of age constituted 25% of all users of anti-anxiety and sedative drugs.
*Fleming & Cross	1:3	
Bass and Baskerville (1981)	more women	Prescribing related to higher frequency of visits, previous tranquilliser use and being female.
Williams et al (1982),Clare and Williams 1981)	-	A proportion of women who complained of depression received tranquillisers rather than anti-depressants which the men in the sample received.
*Varnum (1981)	more women	A higher proportion of men than women are not given psychotropic therapy for a psychological problem.
Williams (1983)	1:1.5	Typical patient at risk is a woman, previously treated with psychotropic medication, with social problems, and with current psychotropic drug treatment of over four months.

Literature Summary 3 cont.

Mellinger & Balter (1981)	1:2	14% of women and 7.5% of men used a medically prescribed anti-anxiety agent in the year prior to interview.
Murdoch (1980)	more women	
Skegg et al (1977)	1:2	7.4% of men and 15.8% of women received sedatives or hypnotics during one year. 9.7% of men and 21% of women received at least one psychotropic drug during one year.
Ingham (1981)	-	Women are more likely than men to consult the doctor for psychological symptoms.

* psychotropic drugs in general, rather than only benzodiazepines.

3.4 Benzodiazepine consumption in the elderly

Swift (1981) reported that, despite the evidence linking disturbed behaviour in the elderly to psycho-active drug use, nearly 90% of prescriptions for nitrazepam go to patients over 65 years of age. Given the evidence that sleep patterns change naturally with age, teaching the patient to expect disturbed or reduced sleep at night could be sounder practice than dispensing hypnotics.

Fleming and Cross (1984) reported that patients over 65 received one third of all psychotropic drugs prescribed in their practice, and, in the American survey of Mellinger and Balter (1981), the maximum use of anti-anxiety agents was in the age group 50-64 years, and that of hypnotics in the group 65-79 years. (Literature summary 4). A study by Purpura (1981), evaluating hypnotic use, commented that 25% of all hypnotics prescribed are consumed by geriatric patients. Presumably the

prescriptions are primarily to aid the management of elderly patients
rather than in response to psychological disturbance per se: Bass and
Baskerville (1981) reported that no association was found between age and
the prescribing of minor tranquillisers for emotional problems, indicating
that the main age difference is the increased use of hypnotics.

Literature summary 4
The use of benzodiazepines in various age groups

Author	Age group	Comments
Mellinger & Balter (1981)	50-64	Maximum use of anti-anxiety agents.
	65-69	Maximum use of hypnotics
*Fleming and Cross (1984)	over 65	Received 33% of all psychotropic drugs prescribed.
Bass & Baskerville (1981)	-	No association between age and prescribing for emotional problems.
Purpura (1981)		Geriatric patients consume 25% of all hypnotics prescribed.
Swift (1981)	over 65	Nearly 90% of prescriptions for nitrazepam go to patients over 65 years of age.

*Psychotropic drugs in general rather than only benzodiazepines.

3.5 Class and employment differences in benzodiazepine use

Dunnell's work, published in 1973, reported that a higher proportion of
the working class population consulted for depression or sleeplessness,

but that a higher proportion of the middle class got sedatives. It was questioned whether this resulted from the middle classes communicating their needs more effectively. Later work by Williams (1983) reported rather different findings, such that women with more than two social problems received psychotropic drug treatment for longer than women with only one or no social problems.

Cook et al (1982), reporting on a survey of nearly 8,000 middle-aged men for the British Regional Heart survey, noted that 28% of men who were physically ill and unemployed consumed benzodiazepines. This was 3-4 times the rate of consumption of benzodiazepines of those who were not ill, whether employed or not. Bass and Baskerville (1981) found no association between prescribing of minor tranquillisers for emotional problems and employment status. Thus, it would seem that being ill rather than being unemployed is linked to an increased use of benzodiazepines.

3.6 Reasons for the prescription

A thought provoking survey by Tyrer (1978) of the drugs taken by 287 GP referrals to an out-patient psychiatric clinic revealed that half of the drugs had been incorrectly prescribed on pharmacological grounds. In addition, in a group of 61 patients who had been taking drugs on a regular basis for more than a year, 20 (one third) had initially been prescribed the drugs in the psychiatric clinic and the tablets had been continued for no obvious reason. Similarly, Johnson and Clift (1968) had shown that doctors repeated prescriptions for hypnotics, first issued in hospital, without consideration of the needs of the patient for continuation of the drug.

Parish (1973) pointed out that therapeutics tended to be neglected in courses offered to doctors, and thus the drug representative's patter may be potent in decision making. In interpersonal terms, the prescription may be offered to appear kindly rather than to respond therapeutically to a need (Oswald, 1983). Hemminki (1975) found that doctors' evaluation of psychotropic drug use was related to the social background of the patient, societal demands, colleagues' views and especially the messages from the drug industry, not to a medical or scientific background.

3.7 Repeat prescribing

The benzodiazepines are often given on repeat prescriptions when the patient is not required to see the doctor each time (Literature summary 5). Varnum (1981) found a difference in the average time on psychotropic drug therapy according to whether the patients were seen or not (4.3 years for those not seen, 2.7 years for those seen). Owen and Tyrer (1983) comment that anxiety tends to run a chronic course, so long term benzodiazepine medication is not surprising. However, Varnum's figures suggest that repeat prescribing compounds the problem, leading to longer term use than when the doctor is more closely involved.

Literature summary 5
Repeat prescribing

Author	Method	Results
Fleming and Cross, 1984	Practice activity analysis of 269 doctors	51% of all psychotropic prescriptions were issued as repeats.
Manasse, 1974	Survey of prescribing of 14 doctors	1/3 repeat prescriptions were given for psychiatric disorder. Repeat prescriptions for psychotropic drugs go to 1.1% of the population.
King et al, 1982	GP prescribing data for all practices in Northern Ireland	60% of prescriptions for tranquillisers were issued as repeats
Dennis, 1979	Survey of 13 practices	2/3 of the repeat prescriptions for psychotropics were for benzodiazepines.

Fleming and Cross (1984), in a practice activity analysis of 269 doctors, found that 51% of all prescriptions for psychotropic drugs were issued as repeats. Manasse (1974) in a study of 14 doctors showed that one third of repeat prescriptions were for psychiatric disorder and estimated that repeat prescriptions for psychotropic drugs go to 1.1% of the population. In a survey in Northern Ireland, King et al (1982) showed that 60% of prescriptions for tranquillisers were issued as repeats. Dennis's survey of 13 practices (1979) found that benzodiazepines formed two thirds of the repeat prescriptions for psychotropics. The study also showed that longer repeats went to older patients who were less closely monitored by the GP.

It has been suggested (Melville 1980) that repeat prescribing of minor tranquillisers is linked to a negative view of the patients' emotional problems. The doctor may be able to preserve a high level of job satisfaction by distancing from more difficult patients. Doctors who believe that emotionally disturbed patients genuinely need help, and that they themselves are capable of giving the help, are much less likely to give repeat prescriptions without seeing the patient (Melville, 1980).

3.8 Expectations of patients

Marinker (1973) postulated that doctors can feel helpless when faced with a population of patients expressing an overwhelming need to alter chemically their experiences of the world in which they live. Typically, doctors are trained that they must "do something" when faced with a patient's problem and that offering understanding is not a sufficient response. The prescription may be viewed as a genuine way of helping people, given that the doctor often can do nothing to change the details of the individual's life. Another powerful influence in determining the prescribing behaviour may be the advertising from pharmaceutical companies which tries to persuade the doctor than when feelings of not coping with the patient arise, then the only action possible is the prescribing of tranquillisers for the patient (Cooperstock, 1979).

However, it is the giving of the prescription which strengthens or creates the expectations of patients that there is a chemical solution to their problems (Parish, 1982). The implicit message in the issuing of the prescription is that the chemicals are the treatment for a problem and thus the problem is labelled as medical (Stimson, 1976). Murray et al (1982) found that the majority of patients who had taken psychotropic drugs for more than six months could not conceive of an alternative to their drugs The authors cited Balint et al (1970) who emphasised the link between receiving long-term repeat prescriptions and loneliness, unsatisfactory marriages, a lack of engagement in social activities and a feeling of "not belonging". Whether the problems were evident prior to the prescriptions or were iatrogenic was not stated, but, clearly, long-term drug therapy fails to overcome a number of negative features in individuals' lives.

One crucial outcome of giving prescriptions is that patients find that their capacity to draw on their own reserves is undermined (Catalan and Gath, 1985). The patient may have gone to the GP for advice, or even just a listening ear (Bradley, 1981) but the doctor can over-estimate the patient's expectations of tangible action, particularly of prescribing. In a study by Jones (1979), 70% of doctors thought that antibiotics, tranquillisers, hypnotics and anti-depressants were over-prescribed, and nearly half of their patients agreed. Thus, the doctor's belief that the patient expects, and thus should be given, a prescription is somewhat misguided. Rapoport (1979) reported that prescribing less led to lowered patient expectations of receiving a prescription.

4. DEPENDENCE

4.1 Definitions of dependence

Although there is considerable reference in the literature to the issues of pharmacological versus psychological dependence, in many respects the distinction is unhelpful in understanding the behaviour of individuals taking benzodiazepines. Behaviour resulting from psychological dependence may be indistinguishable from that caused by physical dependence. The World Health Organisation Expert Committee on Drug Dependence (1974) defined drug dependence as a state, psychic and sometimes also physical, resulting from the interaction between the living organism and a drug, characterised by behavioural and other responses that always include a compulsion to take the drug on a continuous or a periodic basis in order to experience its psychic effects, and sometimes to avoid the discomfort of its absence. Thus, their concern was with the behaviour produced by being dependent rather than focussing on distinguishing physical from psychological features of dependence.

However, many workers do differentiate between physical/ pharmacological and psychological dependence. Edwards et al (1984) describe psychic dependence as a condition in which a drug produces a feeling of satisfaction and psychic drive that require periodic or continuous administration of the drug to produce pleasure or to avoid discomfort, whereas physical dependence is defined as an adaptive state that manifests itself by intense physical disturbances when the administration of the drug is suspended.

Rather differently, Owen and Tyrer (1983) comment that in psychological dependence a patient may insist that a tablet is helpful even if given a placebo, whereas psychological dependence with a pharmacological basis leads to active drug-seeking to produce pleasure or to prevent discomfort. With reference to the benzodiazepines, they suggest that pharmacological dependence, with a rapid development of tolerance and a consequent increase in dosage to produce the same effect is not a common feature.

4.2 Tolerance

Tolerance is a term implying changes such that the same amount of the drug when administered over a period of time ceases to produce the same effects, so that larger doses may be needed. There are two major types of tolerance: dispositional or metabolic tolerance caused by changes in metabolism such that the drug is cleared more quickly from the body; and receptor site tolerance which results from an adaptation of the receptor sensitivity.

There is little evidence of escalation of dose of the benzodiazepines (Lader 1981b), most patients maintaining themselves on a fairly constant dose and increasing medication only in response to increased problems and stress. The very few patients who do increase their dosage have often been dependent on other addictive drugs previously. Tolerance is not correlated with withdrawal phenomema (Tyrer and Sievewright, 1984) and often the only indication of dependence is an abstinence syndrome on reduction or cessation of the drug (Tyrer, 1984). Drug taking can be maintained or increased by the pleasurable qualities of the drug or by alleviating unpleasant symptoms on attempted withdrawal of the drug.

4.3 Withdrawal

The withdrawal phase can be conceptualised as a period before the body has adapted to the loss of the drug, when the functions governed by the drug have not yet come under the control of the body. Literature summary 6 shows reporting of withdrawal symptoms from a number of studies. The range of symptoms is broad. Some symptoms clearly demonstrate the antithesis of the action of the drug, for example muscular pain and tremor which are opposed to muscle relaxation, and insomnia which is contrary to sedation. Many of the symptoms are similar to anxiety, for which the drug may have been prescribed initially, and there has been controversy over whether the experienced symptoms represent a true withdrawal reaction. However, the common experience of perceptual disturbance and the more rare occurrence of grand mal epileptic fits suggest that there are features of the withdrawal syndrome which do distinguish it from underlying anxiety (Tyrer, 1984; Lader, 1981b). (Epileptic seizures have been reported in cases where the dosage of the drug was high (de Bard, 1979; Howe, 1980) or where withdrawal of the drug was sudden (Tyrer et al, 1981).) Owen and Tyrer (1983) suggested that both the occurrence of new symptoms and a temporary increase in pre-existing symptoms are indicative of withdrawal. The temporary nature of the symptoms illustrates the process of adaptation of the body to the non-drug state.

It would appear that shorter-acting drugs produce more severe and abrupt withdrawal reactions (Hollister, 1981; Tyrer and Sievewright, 1984). (The term short-acting refers to the length of time of therapeutic effect, which is different from the half-life of the drug.) Oswald (1983) defined the response to cessation of hypnotics as rebound, ie, an increase in REM sleep and a decrease in sleep duration, accompanied sometimes by fears and paranoid ideas. Shorter-acting hypnotics tend to produce more rebound. Although Shader and Greenblatt (1981) concluded that most patients showing a typical withdrawal syndrome had exceeded the standard dose and had taken benzodiazepines for an extended period, Lader (1981b) found no differences in withdrawal between patients taking therapeutic doses and those taking high doses. Lader (1982) demonstrated, in a study of 50 patients taking less than 30 mg diazepam per day (a normal therapeutic dose), that withdrawal reactions were produced when the drug was halved for two weeks and then stopped. Similarly, Ashton (1984) demonstrated withdrawal in a detailed study of twelve patients who had taken therapeutic doses of benzodiazepines for protracted periods of time (range 3-22 years). A number of other studies have shown withdrawal occurring in some or all of patients when drug therapy ceased (eg, Giblin and Clift, 1983; Tyrer et al, 1981; Petursson and Lader, 1981). Symptoms were most pronounced 3-7 days after stopping medication and tended to resolve within 2-4 weeks.

Tyrer et al (1981) linked withdrawal symptoms to a rapid fall in serum levels of desmethyldiazepam, but later work (Tyrer et al, 1983) found no differences between those who experienced withdrawal symptoms and those who did not in terms of the rate of fall of plasma nordiazepam concentrations. (Desmethyldiazepam and nordiazepam are active metabolites of a number of benzodiazepines.) Thus they postulated that other factors must be involved in the production of the withdrawal syndrome. The design of the study allowed an investigation of false withdrawal, as all subjects believed that the drugs were being reduced from the second week of the study, although, for half the patients, reduction occurred after eight weeks. One in five patients experienced some mild symptoms during the period of treatment when the drugs were unchanged. This suggests that psychological factors do play a part in the production of some withdrawal symptoms.

Optimal periods for reduction of drugs have been suggested by various authors. In general, in-patient withdrawal can be shorter than withdrawal regimes in the community: eg, 2 - 4 weeks (Lader, 1981b) in hospital, as opposed to a minimum of 4 - 6 weeks (and often a much longer period of time) with GP patients (Hopkins et al, 1982; Higgitt et al, 1985). Tyrer (1984) considered that fast withdrawal might produce more intense symptoms, but that slow withdrawal would prolong the symptoms. He suggested that withdrawal could be over a period of up to several weeks and that a flexible dosage up to an agreed maximum was useful. In a similar vein, Higgitt et al (1985) concluded that the rate of reduction should be matched to the occurrence of the withdrawal symptoms. They commented that propranolol, a beta blocker which had been tested to relieve symptoms (eg, Tyrer et al, 1981), did not decrease the frequency nor the subjective aspects of the symptoms, but did reduce their intensity.

Literature summary 6
Withdrawal symptoms

A: Lader, 1982.   B: Petursson & Lader, 1981.
C: Tyrer et al, 1981.   D: Winokur et al, 1980.
E: Shader & Greenblatt, 1981.

Withdrawal symptoms	A	B	C	D	E
Perceptual disturbances/hypersensitivity to auditory and olfactory stimuli	+	+	+	+	+
Severe sleep disturbance/insomnia	+	+	+	+	−
Tremulousness/hand tremor	+	+	−	+	+
Nausea/retching/vomiting	+	+	+	+	−
Muscle pain /twitching/stiffness/numbness	+	+	+	−	+
Profuse sweating/hot and cold flushes	+	+	−	+	+
Headache/head throbbing	+	−	+	+	−
Irritability	+	+	−	+	−
Weight loss/loss of appetite	+	+	−	−	+
Anxiety/panic attacks	−	+	−	+	−
Palpitations/tachycardia	−	+	−	−	+
Dysphoria/feeling that death is imminent	−	−	+	−	+
Choking feeling/dry mouth	+	−	−	−	+
Apparent movement of environment/ unsteadiness	+	−	+	−	−
Epileptic seizures	−	+	+	−	−
Agitation	−	−	−	−	+
Constipation/difficulty in urinating	−	−	−	+	−
Difficulty in concentration	−	+	−	−	−
Depersonalization/derealization	+	−	−	−	−
Psychotic reactions	−	+	−	−	−
Death	−	+	−	−	−

4.4 Characteristics of long-term users of benzodiazepines

Although the notion of a drug dependent personality may be rather
old-fashioned, some factors relating to the individual have been shown to
be associated with dependence on benzodiazepines. Previous drug use has

often been reported in studies of individuals dependent on benzodiazepines and a link with previous or current alcohol use has been demonstrated: Clift, in 1972, reported that patients dependent on hypnotics tended to be alcoholic or to have had previous use of hypnotics; Lader (1981b) commented that those with previous histories of drug abuse and alcoholism were more likely to become tolerant to the benzodiazepines and to escalate the dose; Ayd (1979) suggested that dependence was comparatively rare and primarily occurred in cases not only where there was a history of substance abuse but also where the person was emotionally unstable as well; a study of alcoholic out-patients by Rothstein et al (1976) showed abuse or misuse of chlordiazepoxide in 5% of patients. In summarizing the literature, Griffiths and Ator (1980) concluded that the abuse liability of the benzodiazepines was generally low and that those at risk of developing abusive patterns of drug administration had previously abused sedatives or analgesics.

There is some evidence of cross tolerance of the benzodiazepines with barbiturates and alcohol (Greenblatt and Shader, 1974), thus there could be a simple pharmacological explanation of dependence on benzodiazepines through previous dependence on other psychotropic drugs. However, the explanation may concern psychological features of the pattern of drug use based on operant learning principles and habit formation. Higgitt et al (1985) commented that patients with long-term use of benzodiazepines tended to use their tablets rather than other coping strategies in the face of stress. An individual may select a pattern of drug use as an attempt at problem-solving behaviour, and the short-term relief of anxiety or insomnia may serve to perpetuate the drug taking. Whether there needs to be an underlying personality structure making the individual more prone to this kind of action is a moot point.

In a study of withdrawal by Tyrer et al (1983), those who suffered from withdrawal symptoms were characterised by passsive, dependent personality traits, emotional lability, resourcelessness, sensitivity and impulsiveness. Continued prescribing of tranquillisers can confirm the self image of the individual as being perpetually ill or inadequate and dependent on the doctor. Thus the passive-dependent personality traits may develop over a period of time and represent the result of long-term use, rather than being a determining factor in the genesis of dependence.

5. ALTERNATIVES TO BENZODIAZEPINE MEDICATION

5.1 Psychological therapy as an alternative to medication

A number of studies have reported on the effects of counselling or
behavioural therapy in general practice (Anderson and Hasler, 1979;
Ashurst, 1982; Freeman and Button, 1984; Ives, 1979; Koch, 1979;
McAllister and Philip, 1975; Shepherd et al, 1979; Waydenfeld and
Waydenfeld, 1980). In general, the studies show a reduction both in
visits to the doctor and in requests for medication in the post-treatment
period: for example, Ives (1979) demonstrated a 52% reduction in visits to
the surgery and a 37% reduction in prescription requests in the three
months after psychological treatment, maintained one year later; Shepherd
et al (1979) found that 38% of patients who had received help from an
attached social worker stopped taking psychotropic drugs, compared to 25%
of patients in a control group.

In a controlled trial of the relative effectiveness of cognitive behaviour
therapy, anxiety management training and benzodiazepine drug therapy for
GP patients with a primary problem of anxiety, Lindsay et al (1987)
demonstrated that lorazepam produced the fastest and greatest improvement.
However, as the dose of lorazepam decreased over 30 days, the anxiety
increased to just below the level of anxiety of the waiting list controls.
Both groups receiving psychological therapy showed consistent and
significant improvement as therapy progressed. By follow up, three months
later, the group receiving cognitive behaviour therapy were coping best
with their feelings of anxiety.

Thompson (1985) compared drug treatment with 20 mg clobazam at night with
relaxation and with a combination of the treatments. Patients formed
consecutive referrals to psychiatry and all had had symptoms for at least
one month. Over the short term no differences were evident between the
treatments in terms of outcome, all producing some degree of improvement.
In the longer term, differences may have emerged, as found by Lindsay et
al (1987). The lack of advantage of the combined treatment led to
speculation about the possible detrimental effects on learning of the
drug, or the confusion for the patient of relaxation being induced in two
separate ways.

Controlled evaluation of the effectiveness of brief counselling by the GP
compared to drug therapy showed that both were effective but that patients

receiving counselling were more satisfied with their treatment (Catalan et al, 1984; Catalan and Gath, 1985). There was no evidence of increases in smoking or drinking in the group receiving counselling, demonstrating that the patients were not seeking a drug solution. Robson et al (1984) compared the outcome for patients with psychological disorders by either regular treatment by the doctor or behavioural psychotherapy by a clinical psychologist in the practice. Patients treated by the clinical psychologist achieved greater improvement more quickly than the patients receiving the usual intervention. The latter group made more frequent visits to the doctor and consumed more drugs. In terms of cost effectiveness, it was calculated that 28% of the salary of a clinical psychologist could be found from the drug savings alone.

5.2 Changes in patterns of long-term use of benzodiazepines

Awareness of the problems attached to long-term repeat prescribing of benzodiazepines has increased over the last few years, but, as early as 1972, Clift demonstrated that a simple intervention by the doctor could prevent long-term use. Patients who had taken hypnotics for over six weeks were allocated to groups. One group were advised not to take the tablets for long, the other group served as a control. After one year, 8% of the experimental group, compared to 32% of the control group continued taking hypnotics. Hopkins et al (1982) requested 78 patients, who had taken benzodiazepines for longer than three months, to reduce dosage by one quarter of the original dose, weekly, with the intention of stopping taking the tablets. During withdrawal, weekly interviews with the GP were offered to the patients. 58% of patients stopped medication and 17% reduced to less than half their original dosage. At follow-up, 3 - 5 months later, 63% had stopped completely. Thus, an intervention requiring very little time and effort proved to be effective. Similarly, Cormack and Sinnott (1983) showed that a letter from the GP requesting that tablets be reduced or stopped was as effective as group treatment in anxiety management by a psychologist, resulting in 40% success in reducing or stopping medication.

Anxiety management combining physical and mental relaxation with problem solving strategies has been shown to be effective in helping patients to withdraw from benzodiazepines. Teare Skinner (1984) showed that two thirds of patients could stop taking anxiolytics after six sessions of group work; Giblin and Clift (1983) demonstrated that training in relaxation and advice about getting to sleep were effective in helping

33

elderly patients to stop taking hypnotics.

A more recent study evaluating anxiety management and cognitive techniques for labelling withdrawal symptoms as cues for the implementation of coping strategies (Higgitt et al, 1987) demonstrated success in reducing tablet intake. Patients who received treatment in a group rather than on an individual basis using telephone contact showed lower attrition rates and better long term outcome, indicating the beneficial effect of sharing therapy with similar others.

6. SUMMARY

It has been well-established that long-term use of benzodiazepines occurs in over 1% of the population and that it is, in Lader's words, "an expensive waste of effort" (Lader, 1981a). There have been cited various studies which demonstrate the negative effects of the benzodiazepines in terms of impaired performance, particularly in the elderly. Although doctors may have prescribed the drugs initially for what seemed like good reasons, continuation of long-term use is counter-therapeutic.

Whether long-term use necessarily implies dependence is not clear, but the evidence suggests that there is a range of response to discontinuation and that some individuals may be able to stop using the drugs with minimal effort, while others will suffer a typical withdrawal reaction. Studies of the effects of psychological therapy have shown that patients who respond to the therapy have little need afterwards for psychotropic medication, and there is a limited literature demonstrating the effectiveness of anxiety management approaches in helping patients to reduce benzodiazepine medication after long-term use.

AIMS OF THE RESEARCH

The present research was designed to address a number of questions about
the long-term use of benzodiazepines and the potential for stopping
medication with minimal effort. The literature on withdrawal from
benzodiazepine medication tends to focus on the symptoms that patients
experience, giving the impression that withdrawal is difficult. Only a
few studies indicate that a proportion of patients can withdraw with
comparative ease. The present study was devised to test the hypothesis
that many long-term users of benzodiazepines could reduce or stop
medication simply on the instruction of their GPs.

A further stage of the research was to evaluate the impact of a
psychological programme, specifically designed to help patients to
withdraw from medication. This programme comprised training in
psychological methods of dealing with anxiety and withdrawal symptoms.

The study aimed primarily to answer the following questions:
1. To what extent could a brief intervention by a GP effect a
        reduction in tablet consumption?
2. Which intervention would be more effective - a letter or a
        short interview?
3. What patient characteristics would distinguish those
        successful from those unsuccessful?
4. Would there be differences between GP centres in success rates?
5. Would there be differences between the factors leading to the
        initial prescription of benzodiazepines and those which main-
        tained the consumption of the drug?
6. What strategies devised by the patients would lead to success
        in stopping medication?
7. Would a decrease in benzodiazepines be associated with an
        increase in alcohol or tobacco consumption?

For those who participated in group work, the following questions arose:
                a) Could psychological approaches effect a reduction in
                        tablet consumption?
                b) Which components of the psychological therapy would be
                        most useful for the patients?

OUTLINE OF THE STUDY

1. GENERAL PRACTITIONER INTERVENTION

1.1 Population

One of the findings of the previous work is that the average user of
benzodiazepines is not a person who is constantly demanding the attention
of the general practitioners. Rather, the long-term user tends to be
comparatively unknown to the doctor and merely attends the practice to
pick up the next prescription.

The present study was aimed at this rather anonymous population of
patients who take benzodiazepines on repeat prescriptions over a
considerable period of time. These patients may have very little contact
with the doctor, simply picking up their prescriptions at the reception
desk. Many of these patients may have no particular need for the
medication.

1.2 Identification of the sample

Because the individuals may not be particularly well-known to the doctor,
selection was made through records of repeat prescriptions. Often the
receptionists were the people in the practice who could identify the
patients, and monitoring of repeat prescriptions was performed by the
reception staff. A list of criteria for the selection of suitable
patients for the study was given to the practice and the doctors and
receptionists identified the sample.

1.3 Criteria for selection of the patients

1. The patient had been taking benzodiazepines for at least one
        year.

2. The doctor had no reason to believe that the patient was in
        particular need of benzodiazepine medication at the time.

3. The patient had not been referred to a psychiatrist or

psychologist within the previous two years.

4. The patient was not taking benzodiazepines for epilepsy.

5. The patient was under 65 years of age.

6. The patient did not have a known alcohol problem.

The criteria were developed from the previous study. At the outset, the research intended to evaluate simple interventions which could be useful for people who were taking benzodiazepines as a matter of routine rather than in response to current crisis or illness. Also, the study intended to evaluate psychological approaches with patients who were unfamiliar with the techniques. Thus, excluding those recently referred to psychiatric or psychological services helped to ensure these features. It also prevented the complication of someone outside the practice controlling medication or suggesting changes.

Previous work with the elderly had shown a poor response to interventions by the doctor and difficulty in learning psychological techniques of anxiety management (Cormack and Sinnott, 1983), so those patients over 65 years of age were excluded. However, work published after the start of the project had demonstrated that patients over 70 years of age can be weaned off hypnotics by learning relaxation procedures (Giblin and Clift, 1983).

The hazards of alcohol are potentially greater than those of benzodiazepines, and if reduction of benzodiazepines resulted in an increase in alcohol consumption, then this would be undesirable. The design of the project was such that interventions were purposely minimal; a patient who was likely to increase alcohol consumption would need more intensive work from the doctor than was to be provided within the context of the research project. However, this is not to suggest that doctors should not work to assist patients to reduce consumption of both alcohol and benzodiazepines, particularly as the combination is highly undesirable when operating machinery or driving motor cars.

1.4 The practices

The practices were selected from a list of practices where the doctors had expressed an interest in the research and a desire to participate. Some of the doctors had attended a talk given to the Merseyside and North Wales Faculty of the Royal College of General Practitioners, where a paper had been presented on previous research on the area (Cormack, 1981a). A number of doctors in the audience were interested in becoming involved in the current project. Others knew about the research through personal contact. Practices were selected which were within reasonable travelling distance of the author's (MC) base.

1.5 The experiment

Having selected a sample of patients from a number of different practices, a controlled experiment was set up to compare two interventions from the GP: a letter sent to the patient or an interview conducted in the practice. Thus an evaluation could be made of their comparative success, controlling for any media impact by having a group who received no intervention. By using a number of practices, the effects of any individual doctor would be minimized and the results could generalise more widely.

1.6 Allocation of patients to groups

Within each practice there were three groups:
- a) one group received a letter from the doctor;
- b) one group received an interview from the doctor;
- c) one group had no intervention for a six months monitoring period.

As far as was possible, a rough matching of groups according to age and sex was achieved, but beyond this, patients were randomly allocated to groups. Patients who were near-neighbours or were known to be friends or acquaintances were placed in the same group so that they would not be confused by accounts of different approaches, should they discuss the intervention. Given the comparatively small numbers it was not possible to match for type of tablet, duration of use or size of dose.

1.7 Interventions

a) Letter

Following the success in a previous study of a simple letter in achieving medication reduction (Cormack and Sinnott,1983), doctors were asked to send a letter to patients asking them to cut down on the tablets they were taking. The letters were designed to be non-anxiety provoking and made it clear that prescriptions would not be stopped by the doctor. Advice was given to the patient to cut down gradually rather then stopping abruptly. An example of the letters sent is given below.

Letter from practices

Dear

Recently, experts have begun to worry about people taking tranquillisers for long periods of time. Tranquillisers are only meant to be taken for a short time while you are under stress. Once a crisis has passed the idea is to stop them, not to continue for months or years. Over a long period of time, the body gets so used to the tablets that it does not work properly without them. This means that if you stop taking the tablets you may experience unpleasant withdrawal symptoms for a while until the body gets used to coping without the tablets. We would like you to reduce the number of tablets you take because we believe you would be better without them now. Usually it is best to cut down very gradually over a few weeks so that you will avoid the possibility of experiencing withdrawal symptoms which may be unpleasant.

To start with, instead of taking them at certain times every day, which can just get to be a habit, we want you to move over gradually to taking them only when necessary. This might mean, for example, that you only take a tablet when there is something you have to do which you know will be difficult for you. Also, if you know that you are going to have a couple of drinks then you should not take a tablet.

What we want you to do is to see how long you can make this

batch of tablets last. We will make a note of the day you were
given the prescription and the day you come back for a repeat.
See if you can make each prescription last for a longer time
until you are only taking a tablet on odd occasions when you are
having difficulty in coping.

We believe this will be better for you in the long run, so we
would be happier if you try this new idea instead of us having
to go on giving you tablets month after month.

Yours sincerely

b) Interview

The doctor was asked to interview the patient and to cover the
following points:
1. Explain the doctor's concern about the long-term use of
      benzodiazepines;
2. Advise the patient to cut down gradually;
3. Advise on specific problems if requested;
4. Reassure the patient that the tablets would not be stopped;
5. Tell the patient that prescriptions would be monitored to see
      what progress was achieved.

There were differences between practices in the method of inviting the
patient to interview. The patient was sent an appointment to see the
doctor. If the appointment was failed, a note was attached to the record
indicating that no repeat prescription could be given until the patient
had seen the doctor. Otherwise, a note was issued with a prescription
asking the patient to arrange to see the doctor before the next
prescription was issued. In some cases the doctor took the opportunity to
conduct the interview when the patient happened to attend for a
consultation.

c) Control

The patients in the control group received no communication from the
doctor about their medication. Their prescriptions were monitored over
the six months following the sending of the letter to those in the letter
group. This timing was designed to control for any major impact from the

media which might have led to a general reduction in drug consumption. Once the control group had been monitored for six months, they were to be offered the intervention which the doctors preferred.

1.8 Calculation of tablet equivalence

Because of the variations in the characteristics of the benzodiazepines and the inter-individual differences in rates of absorption and elimination, any attempt to equate them proved difficult. After much consideration and discussions with a pharmacist colleague, a calculation of equivalence was made. Diazepam 5 mg was taken as representing one tablet and equivalents were calculated according to the recommended dosage cited by the manufacturers in the current MIMS, e.g. 5 mg diazepam = 1 mg lorazepam = 5 mg nitrazepam.

2. INTERVIEW WITH THE PSYCHOLOGIST

After the six month monitoring period, patients were invited to attend for interview with the author (MC) to discuss their progress and their strategies for reducing medication. The interviews took place in the practices and were arranged at times convenient to the patients, as far as possible. Details of the reasons for taking the medication and changes in use over time were collected, along with information on consumption of the tablets and smoking and drinking behaviour.

3. GROUP WORK IN PSYCHOLOGICAL ALTERNATIVES

If patients wanted extra help to reduce medication, they were offered the chance of joining a group within the practice to learn psychological approaches designed to deal with anxiety and withdrawal symptoms. The structure and content of the sessions evolved from previous group work with patients who were trying to stop benzodiazepine medication (Cormack and Sinnott,1983).

3.1 Contracts

At the first meeting of the group, stress was placed on the importance of regular attendance and completion of homework tasks. It was made clear that progress could only occur if the participants followed the planned programme and it was indicated that homework tasks would be discussed in the group. Attendance at the group was portrayed as important because group members relied on each other and non-attendance would affect others in the group. Patients signed a written agreement to attend the group.

3.2 Duration of the group

The group was planned for eight weeks with a follow-up session six weeks later. Each meeting lasted for one hour followed by half an hour of tea and chat for the participants without the therapist present. This design allowed for structured work to be the focus of the first hour followed by a half-hour giving the participants a chance to share problems and exchange useful tips on reducing medication.

3.3 Content of group work

a) Education

Emphasis was placed on understanding the clinical effects of the benzodiazepines, and the possible withdrawal effects that might be experienced. In the first two sessions the majority of time was devoted to information giving. A hand-out was used which explained about anxiety, the use of benzodiazepines and approaches to stopping medication.

b) Physical relaxation

Training in relaxation was introduced in the second session with the therapist demonstrating progressive muscle relaxation exercises. Homework tasks were to practise for 20 minutes each day at home, either by listening to the therapist's voice on tape instructing in the exercises, or by following a written sheet with the same sequence of exercises. The psychologist explained the rationale for physical relaxation and stressed that mental relaxation would be tackled as a second stage in the process of relaxing. Subsequent sessions began with relaxation and checked how the homework relaxation task was progressing for each member.

c) Breathing exercises

Because it is commonly found that anxious people have a tendency to hyperventilate (Ley, 1985; Rapee, 1985), a breathing exercise was taught which focused on breathing out and relaxing the chest muscles. A modification of the approach was introduced which could be used unobtrusively at times when the individual could feel tension rising.

d) Self-monitoring

Increasing self-awareness of when tension arose could be useful in activating tension-reduction strategies. Tasks included: rating tension on a ten-point scale on the hour, every hour; becoming more aware of physical tension by practising relaxation exercises; recognising when the mind was racing; noting antecedents of increased tension.

e) Cognitive restructuring

This approach follows from the assumption that what people say to themselves in the form of internal speech, and how they evaluate and interpret events, are modifiable (Meichenbaum, 1977). Aspects of the therapy include education in the role of cognitions in contributing to the current problem and encouragement of positive self-evaluation and coping skills.

Subjects were taught the following strategies: changing negative to positive statements, learning self-reward, slowing the pace of thoughts, focusing on what had been achieved rather than on what was still undone, goal-setting, planning, learning to do things in small steps, giving realistic assessments of what was happening rather than turning events into seeming catastrophes, facing anxiety/problems squarely and not avoiding difficulties.

3.4 Homework tasks

1. Every week a daily diary of number of tablets taken was completed and brought to the group.

2. Relaxation exercises were to be practised at least once daily

until mastered, when the individual could progress to quick relaxation, where all parts of the body are relaxed by mentally monitoring tension and relaxing muscles without having to tense them first. Usually this is done in conjunction with imagining a relaxing scene. The daily routine had to be altered to make relaxation a positive aspect of the day's activities.

3. Breathing exercises were to be practised three times per day until mastered and then used regularly.

4. Various monitoring tasks were set such as tension rating, giving oneself a running commentary on tension in various parts of the body, noting situations where anxiety was high or low, attending to one's own thoughts and recognising how panic arises.

5. Cognitive therapy tasks to increase positive thoughts and self esteem were set. At night time, subjects listed the good things that they had done or that had happened to them that day. At mid-day, subjects looked back over their self-statements and changed any negative ones to more positive and realistic statements.

6. Self-reinforcement was taught by breaking a task into small, easily tackled steps, attempting the first step and, if successful, reinforcing with a predetermined appropriate reward. Rewards were often relaxing and pleasant activities such as going out with a friend or spending some time reading a favourite book.

3.5 Tablet withdrawal

The therapist set limits on the speed of tablet reduction, encouraging participants not to attempt to cut down too quickly. However, the subjects were allowed to go as slowly as they liked. Tyrer and Sievewright (1984) suggested that withdrawal over 6-8 weeks was optimal; Higgitt et al (1985) indicated that gradual withdrawal with steps of between 0.5 and 2.5 mg diazepam (or an equivalent in dosage) should be recommended. Dosage was reduced by one eighth, if possible, or one sixth for the first steps of withdrawal. The patient was asked to remain on the first step of withdrawal until he or she felt settled on that dosage and a minimum time for each step was set at one week. Wherever possible, smaller dose tablets were substituted after the first steps so that reduction could continue as gradually as possible.

3.6 Application of strategies

Symptoms of withdrawal were monitored and coping strategies suggested as an alternative to increasing dosage again. Group support often helped the individual to remain on the lowered dose. Patients were taught delaying tactics such that when they needed tablets they would delay for a period of time, initially two minutes, during which time they would practise a coping strategy. If at the end of the time they no longer needed the tablet, then they would wait until they did and again delay for a period. If this strategy was successful, then they gradually increased the delaying period of time. Thus the patients practised alternatives to medication at times of need.

4. SUMMARY

A sample of long term users of benzodiazepines was identified and divided into three groups. One group received a letter from the GP asking them to try to reduce their medication. Another group had a short interview with the GP where they were requested to reduce medication. The third group had no intervention. After six months the control group were sent the letter from the GP and the subjects in the experimental groups were invited to discuss their progress with the psychologist conducting the study.

The aim of the interview with the psychologist was to uncover factors relating to outcome in order to develop predictors of success in reducing medication. Patients who required further help were offered group treatment along cognitive-behavioural lines.

RESULTS

1. SUBJECTS

1.1 Characteristics of subjects and practices

Seventy-eight subjects were selected and allocated to groups. Any
subjects who failed to meet the inclusion criteria at a point after
selection were excluded from the data analysis from that time onwards.
Three patients were excluded from analysis within the first six months:
(a) One patient in the control group was unwittingly requested to stop
medication by another GP in the practice and thus could not be classified
as a control subject any longer. (b) Two subjects (one in the control
group and one in the letter group) were referred to psychiatrists. In
both cases the GPs considered that the need for the referral arose from
circumstances unconnected with the request to stop taking benzodiazepines.

The following data do not include these three subjects at any point in
time, and thus refer to a total of 75 patients, 12 men and 63 women, a
ratio of M:F 1:5.

1.2 Age of the sample

TABLE 1

Age (years)	Number of subjects
Less than 30	1
30 - 34	2
35 - 39	4
40 - 44	9
45 - 49	17
50 - 54	12
55 - 59	16
60 - 64	10
65 and over	4
	75

The median age of the sample was 51 years.

The original maximum age had been set at 65 years, but four patients were included who were older, because their doctors felt that they would be suitable for the study. Forty-five patients (60% of the sample) were aged between 45 and 59, and only one patient was below age 30 years.

2. MEDICATION

TABLE 2
Tablets taken by subjects

Drug	Number of subjects
diazepam	31
lorazepam	9
oxazepam	8
nitrazepam	4
chlordiazepoxide	3
temazepam	3
clorazepate	3
flurazepam	1
medazepam	1
chlordiazepoxide with clidinium bromide	1
diazepam + nitrazepam	3
diazepam + flurazepam	2
diazepam + alprazolam	1
diazepam + temazepam	1
diazepam + clobazam	1
diazepam + lorazepam	1
lorazepam + nitrazepam	1
lorazepam + temazepam	1
	--
	75

The most widely prescribed drug was diazepam, 40 patients (over half the sample) receiving the drug either alone or in combination with another benzodiazepine. Lorazepam was the next most popular prescription, followed by oxazepam. Table 2 shows the breakdown of the numbers of subjects taking each drug (or each drug combination). Eleven of the 75 subjects were taking two benzodiazepines, usually diazepam plus one other.

The preponderance of diazepam in this study is fairly typical: in 1977, Skegg et al reported that diazepam was given to 6.1% of all people in the population. Combining one benzodiazepine with another is not necessarily pharmacologically sound: a daytime tranquilliser may be given to combat rebound anxiety from a short-acting hypnotic (Morgan and Oswald, 1982); however, a change from the hypnotic would be a more useful solution if the anxiety were recognized as iatrogenic.

2.1 Duration of medication

The duration of drug taking was assessed by reference to the medical records. Medication was not continuous in all cases, but duration of use was assessed from the time of the first prescription. Prior to benzodiazepine medication, several subjects had received barbiturates, but only benzodiazepine drugs were taken into account in assessing duration. Most patients had taken more than one form of benzodiazepine over time, either singly or in combination with other benzodiazepines or other psychotropic drugs.

The median duration of drug taking was 12 years, with a third of the sample having taken the drugs for more than 15 years.

2.2 Baseline number of tablets

Prescriptions were noted from the records for the year prior to the start of the study. The range of tablet equivalents taken in the baseline year was 108 to 1,536, with a median of 540. This median figure represents just over ten tablets per week, which is a comparatively small average compared to recommended prescribing levels. However, Tessler et al (1978) found that 45% of people taking diazepam reduced their dosage over time, so this level of consumption may be typical.

There were no significant differences in mean baseline tablet equivalents according to age or sex. To compare duration of use with number of tablets taken, the subjects were divided into three equal categories according to baseline consumption as follows:

low: 108 – 390 tablets per year
medium: 390 – 672 tablets per year
high: 672 – 1,536 tablets per year

Those in the low category had a mean duration of use of 10 years, as
compared to 13 and 14 years for those in the medium and high categories
respectively. It is interesting that, although the differences reached
statistical significance ($F=4.99$ [2,71 df] $p<.01$), there is little
practical significance of the finding. The shorter mean duration of 10
years is still much longer than the recommended duration of use of the
drugs which is normally for a few days or weeks.

3. THE PRACTICES

Description of the practices

Five practices contributed to the study. They were within an urban
geographical area and were within the lower socioeconomic spectrum in
terms of catchment areas. All practices were involved in undergraduate
medical teaching and all had more than one doctor working in the practice,
either as a group, sharing patients, or in partnership with separate
lists.

Practice A was in a health centre in a lower middle class area and trained
general practitioners (14 patients).

Practice B was in a working class area (16 patients).

Practice C was in a deprived working class area (14 patients).

Practice D was in a health centre in a lower middle class area and was
involved in training general practitioners. The doctors operated a policy
of seeing patients every three months for renewal of repeat prescriptions
(20 patients).

Practice E was in a working class area (11 patients).

There were no significant differences among the practices in terms of age of patients, duration of drug use or baseline mean tablet equivalents.

4. GROUPS

4.1 Allocation of subjects to groups

Within each practice patients were allocated to letter, interview or
control group, with a rough matching for age and sex. When the number of
subjects did not equally divide into three groups, the control group
tended to have the smaller number of subjects. Thus the final allocation
of patients to the groups was:

Letter:	29 subjects
Interview:	24 subjects
Control:	22 subjects

4.2 Differences among the groups

No significant differences between groups were found in mean age, gender
or in mean duration of drug use. When the baseline drug consumption was
categorised into low, medium or high, it could be seen that the control
group contained a higher proportion of people in the low category.

TABLE 3
Baseline drug consumption by group

Baseline Consumption	Group			
	Letter	Interview	Control	
Low	7	5	13	25
Medium	10	12	3	25
High	12	7	6	25
	29	24	22	75

Chi squared = 1.74 (4 df)   p < .02

It may have been that, unknown to the psychologist, the doctors biased the allocation of patients to groups by putting those who were higher consumers into the groups who would receive the intervention immediately rather than into the control group where they would wait for six months.

4.3 Allocation of control subjects to intervention group

After six months of monitoring prescriptions, the patients in the control group were given the intervention which had proved most successful within the practice. For all practices, this was the letter.

Two patients did not receive a letter:

a) One patient had received no prescriptions during the monitoring period. It was discovered that she shared her prescriptions for hypnotics with her husband when they went camping. There had been no request for tablets as monitoring took place over the winter months. As it was impossible to know how many tablets would be consumed by the patient, as opposed to her husband, no letter was sent.

b) One patient was deemed by the GP to need her tablets at the time the letter was sent and so was excluded from the intervention.

Two control patients received letters from the doctor at the appropriate time, but left the practices before the six months monitoring was complete. In both cases, the doctors were sure that the letter had not prompted the move. These two patients were therefore excluded from data analysis of the effect of the letter.

Thus, only 18 of the 22 control group patients were included in the letter group, leaving a final total of 71 subjects, 47 receiving a letter, 24 receiving an interview.

SUMMARY

Subjects were predominantly female, representing a range of ages but mostly in the middle-aged category. They were taking a variety of benzodiazepines, with diazepam as the most widely used drug, and were very long-term users. The only difference between the control group and the experimental groups was that those with low consumption tended to dominate the control group.

5. ANALYSIS OF CHANGE OVER TIME IN DRUG TAKING

To look at change over time, the subjects were divided into three equal
sized groups of low, medium and high rates of tablet consumption in the
year prior to the doctor's intervention (baseline) and then looked at
after six months, one year and two years with respect to the same
categories. Statistical analysis of change over time was performed using
Chi squared tests for symmetry.

This statistical design was employed rather than an approach looking at
differences in average consumption rates before and after intervention to
allow for a clearer picture of the numbers of people who reduced. Given
the vast range of baseline tablet consumption, it would have been possible
for a statistically significant difference to be caused by a few high
users reducing consumption substantially, or by a consistent but small,
and clinically insignificant, change. The Chi squared for symmetry
analysis clearly shows when people move from one category to another and
thus presents a visual picture of the trends.

TABLE 4

		After		
		Low	Medium	High
	Low	A	C	C
Before	Medium	B	A	C
	High	B	B	A

In the above table the subjects falling in cells marked A demonstrated no
change in their drug consumption. Subjects in cells marked B showed a
reduction in drug intake, and those in cells marked C showed an increase
in consumption.

In the following tables the reader will note a large number of 0 values in the cells marked C, indicating that few people increased their tablet consumption to a higher category.

5.1 Control group

TABLE 5

Baseline Consumption	Consumption in the first six months			
	Low	Medium	High	
Low	13	0	0	13
Medium	0	3	0	3
High	0	0	6	6
	13	3	6	22

There was no change in the control group – the group who had no intervention. If there had been change, then the figures for the intervention would have had to be corrected to account for an expected change in a particular direction. However, the following figures now stand as being representative of the effect of intervention, unbiased by other factors.

5.2 Intervention groups

The following tables represent changes over time for patients receiving the letter and the interview (71 subjects).

5.2.1 Changes over the first six months

Letter Group
TABLE 6

Baseline Consumption	Consumption in the first six months			
	Low	Medium	High	
Low	17	0	0	17
Medium	6	4	2	12
High	6	3	9	18
	29	7	11	47

Chi squared for symmetry = 12.20 (2df) p<.01

Interview Group
TABLE 7

Baseline Consumption	Consumption in the first six months			
	Low	Medium	High	
Low	5	0	0	5
Medium	8	2	2	12
High	1	1	5	7
	14	3	7	24

Chi squared for symmetry = 9.33 (2df) p<.01

Intervention (letter or interview)

TABLE 8

Baseline Consumption	Consumption in the first six months			
	Low	Medium	High	
Low	22	0	0	22
Medium	14	6	4	24
High	7	4	14	25
	53	10	18	71

Chi squared for symmetry = 21.0 (2df) p<.0001

TABLE 9

Comparison of letter and interview groups on changes in tablet consumption in the first six months

Group	Consumption			
	Decreased	Same	Increased	
Letter	15	30	2	47
Interview	10	12	2	24
	25	42	4	71

Chi squared = 1.30 (2df) p>.05, ns

From the above tables it can be seen that both the letter and the interview were effective in reducing tablet consumption over the first six months after the intervention.

There were no differences between those who received the letter and those who had an interview with the doctor in terms of movement among high, medium and low categories of drug consumption. Only four subjects increased tablet taking, whereas 25 subjects reduced to a lower category.

5.2.2 Comparison of baseline with months seven to twelve of monitoring

Sixty patients were followed up to a year after receipt of the doctor's letter or interview.

Intervention (letter or interview)
TABLE 10

Baseline Consumption	Consumption in months seven to twelve			
	Low	Medium	High	
Low	15	0	0	15
Medium	19	4	0	23
High	7	7	8	22
	41	11	8	60

Chi squared = 33.0 (2df) $p < .0001$

Comparing consumption over months seven to twelve with baseline consumption, a significant reduction was evident. No subjects increased their drug consumption.

5.2.3 Comparison of baseline with consumption in the second year

Thirty-six patients were monitored over the two years after intervention. Because of the staggering of the start of the project over the practices, there were limited numbers of patients who were into their second year after intervention by the end of the data collection period.

<u>Intervention</u> (letter or interview)

TABLE 11

Baseline Consumption	Consumption in the second year			
	Low	Medium	High	
Low	9	1	0	10
Medium	7	4	1	12
High	10	2	2	14
	26	7	3	36

Chi squared = 14.8 (2df) p<.001

Of those who provided data after two years, a significant reduction in tablet consumption from baseline can be observed in the second year after intervention.

Expected frequencies in the cells were low and the results must be interpreted cautiously. However, ten patients with a high baseline consumption and seven patients wth a medium consumption at baseline fell into the low category in the second year, and only two patients showed an increase in consumption.

6. <u>OCCURRENCE OF MAJOR CHANGE</u>

Because the change in tablet consumption was highly significant within the first six months, it is difficult, from the previously presented figures, to know whether the reduction was merely maintained after the first six months, or whether further reduction occurred. The levels suitable at baseline for the low, medium and high categorisations were no longer appropriate as too many people were now in the low category. Thus, a new categorisation was performed by dividing the subjects into three roughly equal groups according to the extent of their consumption during the first six months after intervention. (Low consumption was less than 236 tablet equivalents per year, medium consumption was 236-444 tablets and the high consumption category was more than 444 tablet

57

equivalents per year.) The range of consumption during the first six
months after intervention was from 0 (8 cases) to 1,680 tablets. The
categories of consumption in the first six months after intervention were
then compared with the consumption figures for the following six months
and for the succeeding year. Comparison was also made of months seven to
twelve after intervention with the succeeding year, using the same
categorisation.

6.1. Changes over the second six months

Intervention
TABLE 12

Consumption in the first six months	Consumption in months seven to twelve			
	Low	Medium	High	
Low	16	0	1	17
Medium	8	11	2	21
High	3	4	15	22
	27	15	18	60

Chi squared = 9.67 (2df) p<.01

Thus, there was a significant reduction in tablet taking over the second
six months of monitoring, compared to consumption in the first six
months.

6.2 Comparison of consumption in months seven to twelve with the second year of monitoring

Intervention (letter or interview)

TABLE 13

Consumption in months seven to twelve	Consumption in the second year			
	Low	Medium	High	
Low	16	1	0	17
Medium	4	1	4	9
High	2	2	6	10
	22	4	10	36

Chi squared = 4.47 (2df) p>.05, ns

There was no statistically significant reduction in consumption between months seven to twelve and the second year of monitoring in terms of category of consumption.

Thus the major change in drug-taking occurred during the first year after the intervention from the doctor. This may reflect the fact that people were advised to cut down gradually and thus were continuing to reduce after several weeks or months.

7. FACTORS RELATING TO SUCCESSFUL DRUG REDUCTION

When reducing drug consumption, success may be viewed in various ways but should represent a substantial reduction from baseline, maintained over a period of time. Two categories of success were delineated:

a) Complete success (16 patients: 14 women, 2 men), meaning that the patient had no prescriptions for benzodiazepines during the last year of monitoring.

b)   Partial success (6 patients: all women), meaning that the
      patient had prescriptions totalling less than 100 tablets in
      the last period of monitoring. Patients in this category were
      either taking very few tablets (an average of less than two
      tablets per week) or had stopped completely but had not been
      monitored for a full year after stopping.

Thus, 22 patients, roughly 30% of the sample, were able to reduce
consumption to zero or less than 100 tablets per year.

7.1 Differences between the successful subjects and those not successful

There were no differences in terms of age or group between those
successful and those not successful.

TABLE 14
Success in stopping tablets by practice

	Practice						
	A	B	C	D	E		
Successful	7	5	5	3	2		22
Not successful	5	10	9	16	9		49
	12	15	14	19	11		71

Fisher's exact test   p = 0.14

Although the differences between practices in success rates did not reach
statistical significance, it is worth commenting on trends. It had been
expected that Practice D, with its policy of reviewing prescriptions every
three months, might be less successful as they may already have prevented a
number of users continuing. This practice had less than one third of
subjects stopping medication in camparison to Practice A with more than
half of the subjects being successful. The doctors in Practice A had been
involved in previous similar research with a difference sample of patients
(Cormack and Sinnott, 1983) and may have been more confident in their
approaches, thus having a greater influence.

7.2 Other factors related to success

Success in stopping tablets was not related to duration of use of the drug. However, this finding is set in the context of a median duration of drug use of 12 years. Thus, it cannot be assumed that duration would be unrelated to ability to stop in people who are short-term users.

Subjects who were successful in stopping tablets had a lower mean baseline tablet consumption: 488 tablets per year, compared to 650 tablets for the unsuccessful ($t=2.23$, 69df, $p<.05$).

TABLE 15
Success in stopping tablets by drug

Drug	Number successful
Diazepam	12
Lorazepam	3
Oxazepam	2
Clorazepate	2
Flurazepam	1
Medazepam	1
Chlordiazepoxide with clidinium bromide	1
Total	22

The type of benzodiazepine taken did not distinguish the successful from the unsuccessful subjects, the distribution of drugs in the successful group being similar to that in the sample as a whole.

It was interesting to note that all the successful subjects were taking only one benzodiazepine as opposed to a combination of two benzodiazepine drugs.

TABLE 16

Success by single or combined benzodiazepines

	Successful	Not successful	Total
Single drug	22	37	59
Combined drugs	0	12	12
	22	49	71

Chi squared = 6.48, 1df, p<.02

8. THE PSYCHOLOGY INTERVIEW

8.1 Numbers of patients attending the psychology interview

Thirty eight patients were interviewed by the psychologist. One of these interviews was conducted over the telephone as the patient had difficulty attending the practice due to work commitments. Two further patients were interviewed by their GP using the interview form. These were patients who had not responded to the request to meet the psychologist but were willing to answer the interview questions when they were posed by the doctor. There were thus 40 patients providing interview data.

8.2 Differences between attenders and non-attenders

No significant differences were found between those who did and those who did not attend the interview with respect to the following variables: age, sex, duration of drug use, baseline number of tablet equivalents, or success in stopping medication.

A significant difference between attenders and non-attenders was found with relation to the type of intervention from the doctor (Table 17). Three quarters (18/24) of those patients who had previously been interviewed by the doctor attended the interview with the psychologist, compared to less than half (22/47) of those who had received the doctor's letter. Thus, it appeared that talking about medication reduction with the doctor made it easier to go to talk to a psychologist about medication.

TABLE 17

Group by attendance at psychology interview

	Letter	Interview	
Attenders	22	18	40
Non-attenders	25	6	31
	47	24	71

Chi squared = 5.18 (1df) p<.05

8.3 Time of day tablets taken

Of those patients supplying information at the interview with the
psychologist, thirteen took the drugs in the day-time and thirteen at
night, with 4 patients taking the tablets at both times. Drugs taken only
at night were flurazepam, temazepam, clorazepate and nitrazepam (once in
combination with diazepam), all of which are intended to be taken at night
However, diazepam and lorazepam, which are marketed as tranquillisers were
more commonly taken at night-time than during the day.

Patients were asked about their reasons for taking tablets when they were
first prescribed and why they continued to take them. The patients' views
of why they took benzodiazepines could differ from the doctors' views.
However, people's beliefs about why they take drugs are probably more
pertinent to an analysis of their continued use of the drugs than are data
from the medical records concerning the doctors' views of the problem,
particularly as these were patients who, to a large extent, were
controlling their own medication through repeat prescriptions.

For twenty of the patients, their reasons for taking benzodiazepines
changed over the years. This implied that the stimulus for the initial
prescription was no longer operating, but it also suggested that other
features led to the maintenance of drug taking, rather than the drug taking
stopping because the need for medication had disappeared. Seven subjects
reported that the major factor in drug maintenance was habit. Eight
patients had taken benzodiazepines initially following a bereavement and
had developed new reasons for continuing to take them. Although no
patients had started taking benzodiazepines for the relief of somatic

symptoms, four patients were citing this as their major reason for continuation of use.

TABLE 18
Reasons for taking tablets

Reason	Initial factor	Maintaining factor
Psychological distress a)	17	15
Insomnia	5	5
Somatic symptoms b)	0	4
Bereavement	8	0
Chronic stress c)	3	5
Physical illness	3	1
Doctor's instruction	3	1
Habitual use	0	7
	39*	38+

* Missing data for one subject.
+ Missing data for two subjects.

a) Included reports of anxiety, depression and emotional problems.
b) Included tension, lacking energy and pain in the abdomen.
c) This was protracted stress most often including looking after sick relatives.

Note: Where patients gave more than one reason for taking medication, the most important reason was selected for the table. A full list of reasons for taking benzodiazepines is given in the Appendix.

8.4 Strategies employed to reduce medication

The strategies described by subjects for reducing medication fell into four broad categories:

1.   Alternative consumption, such as drinking more tea, coffee or fruit juice, eating more or smoking more (only one patient increased smoking). (3 subjects)

2.   Stopping suddenly (this had not been advised by the doctor).
     (7 subjects)
3.   Gradual reduction, achieved by cutting up tablets or increasing
     the interval between tablet taking. (13 subjects)
4.   Gradual reduction plus alternative therapy, such as yoga,
     breathing exercises, relaxation exercises or following advice
     in a leaflet from MIND. (4 subjects)

The most popular strategy employed by subjects was gradual reduction of
tablets.

8.5 Factors linked to successful stopping of medication

Although the psychology interview was not designed as an intervention in
itself, it was found that the author (MC) not infrequently gave advice to
help people who did not wish to join the group for help. Despite
expectations, this had no effect on the success rates of attenders as
opposed to non-attenders.

Statistical analysis was impossible on some of the data from the interview
due to small numbers in various categories. However, there was a tendency
for successful subjects to be taking the tablets at night, and to be using
them for insomnia or out of habit.

It had been thought that certain strategies for reduction would be more
successful than others but there was no clear evidence that strategy
related to success. Six of the eight successful subjects had used gradual
reduction, but so had eleven of the nineteen unsuccessful. Alternative
consumption had not been a successful strategy for the three subjects who
tried it.

8.6 Summary

Althought it had been intended to discover predictive factors for success,
the interview failed to uncover any clear predictors. It was surprising to
find that those who took medication at night showed a slight tendency to be
more successful. The change of use of the benzodiazepines over time was
interesting, suggesting the possibility that some symptoms may have been
produced by the benzodiazepines: Ashton (1984) found that agoraphobia
developed in patients after taking benzodiazepines. It is also somewhat

disturbing to realise that the subjects in this study were effectively self-medicating through their repeat prescriptions for symptoms which had not prompted the initial prescription.

9. GENERAL SUMMARY OF FINDINGS

1. Both the letter and the interview from the GP served to produce reductions in tablet consumption for patients and the interventions were equally effective.

2. Although reduction in consumption continued over varying periods of monitoring (up to two years), the major reduction occurred in the first six months after intervention.

3. 22 out of 71 patients were successful in stopping taking tablets by the criterion of less than 100 tablets in the last year of monitoring (16 patients stopped medication completely).

4. There were no predictors of success identified in terms of age or sex of subject, duration of benzodiazepine use, GP centre, intervention, baseline tablet consumption or type of benzodiazepine. It was noted, however, that all successful cases were taking only one benzodiazepine.

5. Of the 37 patients providing information at interview, roughly half had continued using benzodiazepines for reasons other than those for which the drugs were prescribed.

6. No single strategy offered by subjects for reducing medication proved to be more successful than any other.

10. GROUP PSYCHOLOGICAL THERAPY

10.1 Formation of the groups

An early intention of the research had been to assess the impact of group
anxiety management training after seeing the effect of the doctor's
intervention. It was assumed that several patients in each practice would
wish to have psychological help after their own efforts to reduce drug
consumption.

Patients in the first three practices (A, B and C) in which the research
was undertaken were offered the chance of joining a group. In only one
practice (B) was there sufficient interest for a group to be formed. No
patients in practice C wanted further help from the psychologist. In
practice A, the only patient who wished to have further help had already
undergone a course of anxiety management some few years previously,
similar to that which would have been offered, and had also stopped tablet
taking. Thus it was not seen as appropriate to suggest that she join a
group.

By the time the other two practices (D and E) were at the stage of
possible psychological involvement to assist the patient, the offered help
had been modified due to the lack of interest in group work by the
patients in the other practices, and also due to a change in job location
of the psychologist, which made a weekly commitment in the practice
untenable. Thus, patients in practice D were offered a leaflet about how
to come off tranquillisers and an audio-tape of instructions on how to
learn to relax. One patient took up the offer. In practice E there
existed, at that time, an anxiety management group, run by an occupational
therapist on the premises. Although patients were encouraged to attend,
only one did so.

Given the poor response to the offer of further help, it was decided to
run two groups of out-patients at local hospitals to test the effects of
anxiety management. Recruitment was through the occupational therapy
department serving both hospitals. Patients who had been referred from
psychiatry for relaxation therapy were selected and their psychiatrists
were asked whether it was appropriate for the patients to reduce or stop
benzodiazepine medication. If the psychiatrists agreed, the patients were
invited to an assessment interview with the occupational therapist who was
to be co-therapist in the group work. Any patients who were unduly anxious

or who failed to comprehend the information given about the group work
were excluded. Similarly any patients who could not commit time to a
regular meeting were not invited to the group.

The groups were single sex (one male, one female) as previous work
(Cormack & Sinnott, 1983) had suggested that this might be advantageous in
terms of group cohesion. Two previous groups had been mixed sex, with a
majority of women in each group. It had been felt that discussion was
sometimes difficult when a topic was perceived as relating to one sex. The
women in the group were more able to share their concerns with other women
and, as a result, the men had sometimes felt peripheral. It was thought
that single sex groups might be more comfortable for participants and thus
more productive in terms of tablet reduction.

If there had been enough subjects, it might have been useful to organise
groups according to those who took tablets to help with sleep and those
who used them during the day. Numbers were insufficient to allow this
distinction, also many patients took tablets both for daytime anxiety and
for insomnia.

The psychologist led all groups and was assisted with the hospital groups
by an occupational therapist. Groups lasted for between eight to ten
sessions and follow-up was six weeks after the last group meeting.

10.2 Changes in consumption over the course of the group

Where patients attended their group infrequently, they were excluded from
data analysis as their results could not be said to represent the effect
of the psychological therapy.

In cases where the patient was taking more than one benzodiazepine, the
data on consumption for each tablet were analysed separately, as patients
were always encouraged to reduce only one kind of medication at a time.
If the medication was changed during monitoring, or if an additional
benzodiazepine was prescribed, then the new tablet dose was converted to
the equivalent of the original.

Hospital group X: female
Three out of 5 patients attended sufficiently frequently for their data to
be subjected to analysis, although no follow-up data were available. The

week of duration of the group was correlated with the number of tablets recorded as taken for that week for each patient and subjected to linear regression analysis.

X1 reduced her consumption of lorazepam 1 mg from 6.5 tablets per week to 0 (linear regression r = -0.96, p<.01). She was also taking amitriptyline hydrochloride and propranolol hydrochloride. The consumption of amitriptyline hydrochloride reduced from 2 to 8 tablets per week and consumption of propranolol hydrochloride increased from 18 to 28 tablets per week. (Information on the sizes of these tablets was not supplied.)

X2 was taking lorazepam 1 mg; she did not reduce her consumption during the course of the group, taking between 6.5 and 9.5 tablets per week.

X3 was taking flurazepam and dothiepin hydrochloride. She had chosen to stop the anti-depressant before trying to reduce the hypnotic. During the course of monitoring she reduced from 1050 mg to 125 mg of dothiepin hydrochloride, but remained static at 7 tablets of flurazepam 15 mg per week.

Thus, only one of the two patients who attempted to reduce benzodiazepine medication was successful.

Hospital group Y: male

All of the group (5 patients) attended sufficiently frequently for analysis of their data and follow-up data were available for three of them.

Y1 was taking lorazepam and lofepramine (an anti-depressant). Consumption of lorazepam dropped from 10 mg per week at the start of the group to 8 mg at the end of the group and 3.5 mg at follow-up (linear regression r = -0.94, p<.001). Consumption of lofepramine did not change during the seven weeks of the group, but the patient stopped the tablets at his own instigation between the end of the group and the follow-up.

Y2 was taking diazepam and chlormezanone (a non-benzodiazepine hypnotic). The number of tablets of diazepam 5 mg taken reduced from 6.5 per week to 1.5 per week by the end of the group (linear regression r = -0.92, p<.01). Consumption of chlormezanone 200 mg reduced from 11 to 2 tablets over the course of the group.

Y3 did not reduce his consumption of lorazepam 1 mg, taking between 21 and 18.8 tablets per week over the course of the group.

Y4 was taking diazepam 5 mg and reduced from 7 to 1.5 tablets per week over the course of the group (linear regression r = -0.85, p<.05), but the gains were lost at follow-up when the patient was taking 14 tablets per week. In the time between the end of the group and the follow-up meeting the patient had been dealing with legal issues surrounding his divorce and had taken more tablets in response to this stress.

Y5 was taking lorazepam and temazepam. Consumption of lorazepam 1 mg changed from 14 tablets to 1 per week by the end of the group and to 0 at follow-up (linear regression r = -0.76, p<.05). Consumption of temazepam 20 mg changed from 7 tablets per week at the start of the group to 3.5 by the end of the group and to 0 by follow-up (linear regression r = -0.93, p<.001).

Although this patient was the most successful, the group work alone may not have been the determining factor in the success rate as he began receiving psychotherapy between the end of the group and follow-up. He had been referred for psychotherapy prior to the start of the group but this had not been revealed to the group leaders at the time of selection for the group.

Thus, of the five patients in this group, four were successful in reducing medication during the course of the group. Of the three who provided follow-up data, two had reduced further and one had increased consumption.

GP group B: female

Two of the five patients attended sufficiently frequently to be included in the data analysis.

There was a break of two weeks (after the sixth week of the group) over Christmas and New Year but patients continued monitoring tablets over this break, providing 11 weeks of data collection. All patients reported that Christmas was a stressful time and this was reflected in increased tablet consumption.

B1 joined the group with the intention of learning strategies for coping without tablets but she had no intention initially to reduce tablets. However, she decided to try reducing tablets towards the end of the group.

70

She was taking both diazepam 5 mg and lorazepam 1 mg and chose to reduce
lorazepam first. Thus there was no change in diazepam consumption (17-14
tablets per week), but a significant change in lorazepam intake from 15
tablets to 12 during the course of the group, and to 0 by follow-up
(linear regression r = -0.84, p<.001).

B2 had stopped taking lorzepam 1 mg some while before starting the group
but wished to join the group to help her to maintain the success. During
the course of the group she had 2 tablets and one more in the follow-up
week. Thus she could be construed as successful in maintaining her lack
of medication.

10.3 Summary of changes in other medication

Information about concurrent psychotropic medication and beta-blockers was
obtained to investigate whether a reduction in benzodiazepines was made at
the expense of an increase in other medication to compensate for the loss.
The only evidence of an increase in other drugs was with patient X1 who
increased propranolol hydrochloride (but at the same time also decreased
amitryptiline hydrochloride). For all other subjects, other medication
either remained the same or reduced.

10.4 Summary of outcome of group therapy

Of the eight patients who intended to reduce medication, six were
successful in doing so during the course of the group, although one lapsed
by follow-up. A further two attended frequently, one maintaining freedom
from medication and one successfully reducing anti-depressant medication.

However, these results refer only to those subjects who attended group
sessions sufficiently frequently for analysis of their data to be
meaningful in the context of their receipt of psychological therapy. Five
other patients in the groups had low attendance, and thus could be
construed as not benefitting from the therapy.

There were various reasions given for why people did not fulfil their
contracts of attendance, but dislike of the therapy or lack of motivation
to reduce medication must be considered as possible factors.

10.5 Strategies employed by the group members for tablet reduction

At follow-up, group members were asked what strategies had been most useful to them in reducing tablet consumption. Their strategies were as follows:

1. Relaxation (3 patients): using the breathing technique, relaxing before going to bed instead of taking a hypnotic, imagining a pleasant scene.

2. Delaying tablet taking (2 patients): instead of taking a tablet first thing in the morning, delaying by 15 minutes and discovering the tablet was not needed.

3. Keeping busy as a distraction technique (2 patients).

4. Reducing gradually by dividing tablet into six pieces.

5. Tackling problems instead of avoiding facing them.

6. Group support: going for a walk as a group after the session.

Comment

All of these strategies had been recommended by the group leaders and it appeared that relaxation was particularly useful. However, it must be remembered that the therapist who led the groups collected this information and it might be expected that a bias would operate to give a response in keeping with the instruction taught to the patients.

10.6 Summary

There was a disappointing response to the offer of group therapy within the practices, so two groups were conducted using hospital patients to determine the impact of group therapy. Although a fair degree of success was encountered with subjects who attended sufficiently frequently, the low attendance rate of other subjects may be construed as a rejection of the therapy and thus as a measure of failure.

DISCUSSION

1. SEX-RATIO OF SUBJECTS

In comparison to other studies (e.g., Balter et al (1974), Skegg et al
(1977)), there were fewer men in the sample than would have been expected:
most other work has indicated a ratio of males to females of 1:2, this
sample had a ratio of 1:5. An unpublished study (Deadman, 1984) of a
similar population of GP patients in Mersey Region found a ratio of 1:3,
males to females, of patients having been prescribed benzodiazepines in
one year. Although the preponderance of women in the present study may
have been a chance finding, it may have been related to the selection
criteria. All patients with a known alcohol problem were excluded and
these were more likely to be men (Madden, 1979). Unfortunately, no figures
were kept on the number and gender of subjects who were excluded for this
reason, although it is remembered that there were very few.

2. AGE OF SUBJECTS

Because of the exclusion in this study of the older age group,
comparison with published data on the age distribution of psychotropic
drug use is difficult. King et al (1982) showed that the majority of
hypnotic prescriptions went to the elderly (over 65 years) and to women
aged 45 - 59 years. In the cross-national survey of Balter et al (1974)
women aged 55 years and over represented one quarter of all users of
anti-anxiety and sedative drugs, and the American survey (Mellinger and
Balter, 1981) showed that the maximum use of anti-anxiety agents was in
the age group 50 - 64 years.

In the present study the median age was 51 years and 60% of the sample
were aged 45 - 59 years, thus the sample might be viewed as fairly
representative of the population of users under 65 years of age.

3. BASELINE TABLET CONSUMPTION

The baseline consumption of the sample (average of 10 tablets per week)
indicated that they were not taking the tablets as would normally be
prescribed. This finding compares with that of Tessler et al (1978), in a
survey of diazepam use, where 45% of the sample reported decreased use

over time and only 6 out of 236 reported taking as much as 40 mg of diazepam (equivalent to eight tablets per day in this study).

At interview with the psychologist the patients not infrequently described a pattern of drug-taking such that they took one tablet per day on a regular basis and another if needed. It was a common theme that patients reported that they did not want to have to take tablets and had purposefully reduced the dose.

4. GROUP DIFFERENCES

At the time of allocating patients to control or intervention groups, matching was by reference to age and sex, not amount of drug consumed. Although the control group were not significantly different from the experimental group in baseline mean number of tablet equivalents, there was a higher proportion of patients in the control group taking low doses of benzodiazepines. No change was demonstrated in drug consumption over the control period of six months, but this could be an artefact of the distribution of patients in the categories. If patients in the low dose category reduced consumption, they would still remain in this category and would not be detected by the chi-squared for symmetry analysis. However, the analysis did show that there was no change in the medium and high dose categories, and there is no obvious reason to predict that those who take fewer tablets would be likely to alter their consumption rates. Given that these patients were all long-term users, the indication was that they would continue so. The only new feature in their situation was the increase in publicity about benzodiazepine dependence. Thus it may be concluded that media reports did not affect consumption rates.

5. LOW ATTENDANCE AT THE PSYCHOLOGY INTERVIEW

In the previous research (Cormack and Sinnott, 1983; Cormack, 1981b) it had been found that patients were reluctant to see a psychologist. Informal enquiry by the doctors revealed that there was confusion about what psychologists do and some apprehension about what might happen at the interview. Care was taken in the present research to overcome these problems either by referring to the psychologist as a researcher from the University or by the doctor explaining the role of the psychologist prior to the interview. However, there was still a relatively low response rate to the invitation to attend the interview with the psychologist.

6. LACK OF INTEREST IN GROUP THERAPY

In the original design, it had been assumed that some patients would
respond to the doctor's letter and be able to reduce medication fairly
easily whereas others would find difficulty in cutting down on tablet
consumption and would need additional help. Thus it was anticipated that a
number of people from each practice would be interested in joining a group
to learn alternatives to medication. In the event, very few subjects
volunteered for group work, partly because many subjects said they could
manage without extra help or for various reasons chose not to become
involved in group therapy. Another factor contributing to the low uptake
of the offer of group therapy was the high proportion of subjects who
failed to attend the interview with the psychologist and thus did not
learn about the possible existence of a group.

7. WITHDRAWAL FROM DIAZEPAM AND LORAZEPAM

All of the drugs taken by those who were successful in stopping
tablet-taking were prescribed either for anxiety or for insomnia where
day-time sedation was acceptable (MIMS recommendations). Thus none of the
drugs was short acting, except for lorazepam which does not have active
metabolites . It had been commented that shorter acting benzodiazepines
(particularly lorazepam) would tend to produce more severe withdrawal
reactions (Tyrer and Seivewright, 1984). However, it cannot be concluded
from this study that it was easier to withdraw from diazepam than from
lorazepam, as roughly one third of patients taking each drug were
successful.

8. DIFFERENCES IN SUCCESS WHEN TAKING SINGLE OR COMBINED BENZODIAZEPINES

None of the subjects who took more than one benzodiazepine were successful
in stopping medication. It has already been mentioned that a day-time
anxiolytic may be prescribed because of rebound anxiety caused by a short
acting hypnotic. There was no evidence in the present study to explain
why two drugs were being prescribed, but in the case of combinations such
as diazepam and nitrazepam or diazepam and flurazepam (the most common
combinations), there appears little logic in simultaneously prescribing
two long-acting compounds. The implications of the success rates are that
only one benzodiazepine should be prescribed if dependence is to be
avoided.

9. REASONS FOR THE SUCCESS OF THE DOCTORS' INTERVENTIONS

Some indications of why the intervention should have been successful were given by patients who attended interview. Eight patients had fallen into a habit of taking the tablets, or else felt that the GP wished them to continue medication, and the instruction from the doctor made them re-assess their need for the tablets. Other patients took very seriously the request to cut down or stop the medication and were also aware of the concern about benzodiazepine dependence from the media.

The doctors had all emphasised to the patients that the tablets would be monitored but that the prescriptions would remain available. A few patients expressed worries that the doctors might in time prevent them from having the prescriptions and thought that they ought to reduce consumption before they were forced to do so. This was not the plan in any practice, but the concern about it had an effect.

A number of patients suggested that they did not really want to take benzodiazepines and the letter or interview had been the impetus that was needed for them to start to make changes. In general, a very negative view of drug taking was held by patients and any thought that they might be drug addicts was of considerable concern. Reducing drug consumption was a way of demonstrating that they were not dependent on the drugs.

10. EFFECT OF A DECREASE IN BENZODIAZEPINES ON ALCOHOL AND TOBACCO CONSUMPTION

Only one patient reported an increase in other drug consumption: she had stopped taking diazepam abruptly and doubled her cigarette smoking from 30 to 60 per day. The psychologist advised that she might be safer taking benzodiazepines than smoking so much. No other patients reported an increase in alcohol or tobacco consumption when benzodiazepines were reduced. This parallels Ashton's (1984) finding that none of her subjects replaced benzodiazepines with other drugs or alcohol.

Given the evidence of cross-tolerance of some benzodiazepines with alcohol (Greenblatt and Shader, 1974), it might have been expected that subjects would have sought alcoholic alternatives when deprived of their usual drug. However, this was not the case according to the interview data. It

might be conjectured that the rate of any reduction, being controlle
each individual, was sufficiently slow to prevent craving for alternati
and that the readily available benzodiazepines would have been taken if a
drug were needed. Also, the sample were predominantly women who drank only
occasionally on social outings and so they were most unlikely to
substitute alcohol for the benzodiazepines. (Patients with a known
alcohol problem had been excluded from the study because of the concern
that substitution of one drug for another might occur.)

11. DIFFERENCES BETWEEN THE FACTORS LEADING TO THE INITIAL PRESCRIPTION OF BENZODIAZEPINES AND THOSE WHICH MAINTAINED THE DRUG CONSUMING

For half of the patients who provided information at interview the initial
reasons for the prescription were different from the reasons given for
maintenance of medication. Ashton (1984) had drawn attention to symptoms
which appeared after the start of benzodiazepine therapy, particularly
agoraphobia which developed in 11 out of the 12 patients and improved
remarkably on withdrawal of the drugs. She commented on common symptoms of
prolonged use of benzodiazepines as: loss of concentration and memory,
decline in psychomotor performance, depression and emotional anaesthesia.
Four subjects in the present study reported developing agoraphobia while
taking benzodiazepines, two subjects who were prescribed the drugs for
agoraphobia maintained their use for other reasons and one subject remained
agoraphobic. From the descriptions of symptoms given, it was difficult to
qualify what the changes were over the course of time of taking the drugs,
but the broad category of psychological distress accounted for over one
third of the reasons for continued use. Over one fifth of patients who
provided data at interview cited habit as a factor in maintenance of drug
taking. It was not clear to what extent the term "habit" described true
dependence as opposed to continued use for no specific reason, but three of
the seven patients stopped taking tablets, suggesting that the habit could
be broken.

At a more general level, there was some cause for concern that several
patients were effectively self-prescribing in choosing to use the repeat
prescription for reasons not discussed with the general practitioner. It
is acknowledged that the prescribing of benzodiazepines should be in the
hands of skilled professionals. In particular, if symptoms are due to the
long-term use of benzodiazepines, then continued use, in an attempt to
relieve these symptoms, is inappropriate.

ategies were described and categorised into four groups: no
emerged as being associated with success. Given that
patients in general did reduce their dosage of medication, it suggested
that an intention to reduce was more important than the specific approach
to reduction indicated by subjects or else that different strategies suit
different people. It was interesting to note that sudden stopping of
medication, although it had not been advised by the doctors, was not
significantly less successful that the recommended gradual reduction.

13. EFFECT OF THE GROUP PSYCHOLOGICAL THERAPY ON TABLET CONSUMPTION

Although reductions in tablet consumption were evident in roughly half of
the subjects who joined group psychological therapy, consideration must be
given to factors other than psychological approaches in explaining the
reductions. There was no control group so it was not clear whether
non-specific factors of the group rather than the psychological approaches
per se would have accounted for the observed changes. In all groups there
was a strong expression of the supportiveness of the other group members
and the half-hour of tea and chat was viewed as important.

Future work could benefit from more stringent selection procedures to
assess motivation for therapy and to gain higher attendance at group
sessions.

14. COMPONENTS OF THE PSYCHOLOGICAL THERAPY WHICH WERE MOST
    USEFUL FOR PATIENTS

In support of a positive effect of the psychological therapy was the
feedback from group members about aspects of the group work which were
helpful. Training in relaxation appeared to be particularly useful and
this obviously mimicked the benzodiazepines in muscle relaxant effect.
The breathing exercise was often reported by group members as a useful
activity in between sessions when they felt particularly tense. As this
exercise helped to prevent hyperventilation and thus avoided any

consequent panic feelings, it may have worked directly to reduce the need for medication.

Other strategies which were commonly mentioned were various problem solving approaches. Given that the majority of the benzodiazepines have a detrimental effect on a number of cognitive functions (Lader, 1983a; Hendler et al, 1980), it would be expected that problem solving capacity would be reduced. There could then emerge a circular process of poorer problem solving generating fewer alternative strategies for coping, leading to more need for benzodiazepines, leading to further dulled cognitive functions. Breaking out of this circle by experiences of effective problem solving could be crucial in recognising alternatives to medication and thus reducing tablet taking.

COMMENTS ON THE WORK

1. METHODOLOGICAL CONSIDERATIONS OF THE PRESENT STUDY

1.1 Limitations of the interview data

It was noted that there were missing data for many of the questions posed at interview and that just over half of the subjects attended the interview. Often these omissions may have been unavoidable, for example, most studies suffer some subject attrition. Nonetheless, a different style of introduction of the psychologist and a firmer procedure for ensuring that invitations to interview had been sent might have resulted in more interviews being achieved.

Although the interviewer had been trained in clinical and research interviewing, patients did sometimes divert the interviewer from the line of questioning. To some extent, this might be typical of this population who may be anxious or may be lacking concentration. The interviewer must establish rapport and appear empathetic to the emotional content of the subjects' responses while at the same time pursuing a distinct line of enquiry and attempting to get direct answers to questions. At times the latter task proved too difficult without losing rapport and thus some data were not collected.

1.2 Future expansion of the interview

Predictions of success did not emerge clearly in this study. The interview should be expanded to cover a greater range of questions in an attempt to unearth predictions. Obvious areas of expansion are to gather information on educational attainments and occupation to indicate the general abilities of the person, which may be relevant to finding and utilising alternatives to drug intake. Details of the social and emotional support available to the person at the time of reduction of medication may be pertinent to assessing the success of the attempt to reduce. Some measure of motivation to reduce drug-taking would be useful, although this may be difficult to obtain in the interview if the interviewer is viewed as desiring that the interviewee reduce drugs. A description of the relationship between patient and doctor from both points of view might be a crucial factor in determining compliance with the request to change drug-taking behaviour.

At the interview insufficient evidence was gathered to assess the extent
to which withdrawal symptoms were experienced. A closer investigation of
the patient's experience of attempts to stop benzodiazepine use could
perhaps unearth the nature and severity of withdrawal and link to the
ability to continue drug reduction.

1.3 Control of medication in the hospital groups

Although the referring psychiatrists were clearly informed of the work, a
warning sticker about benzodiazepine prescribing could have been attached
to the medical notes to help prevent the prescription for a different
benzodiazepine (temazepam) which was given to a patient who had been
successful in stopping lorazepam. Patients could also have been encouraged
to enquire whether any new drug prescribed was a benzodiazepine.

2. IMPLICATIONS OF THE STUDY

2.1 Benefits for the patients

The evidence on the detrimental effects of the benzodiazepines on
performance, cognitive and psychomotor, and the limited evidence of brain
damage following long-term use suggest that people may perform better in a
number of ways without the drugs. If the drugs prevent adequate problem
solving, then patients may be caught in a situation of having to continue
drug taking because they cannot find another way of dealing with their
symptoms. Attempts to tackle the causes of the symptoms may not be
initiated or may fail through decreased problem solving skills. Helping
people to cease or reduce benzodiazepine consumption may open up avenues
to other coping strategies. Anecdotal evidence from patients seen by the
author and other workers in the field supports the view that people feel
that their capacities have been dulled by the drugs and that a new or
forgotten self emerges when the drugs are discontinued.

2.2 Cost benefits

In Mersey Region, in 1984, the net ingredient cost of prescriptions for

81

hypnotics, sedatives and tranquillisers issued by Family Practitioner Services was £2,650,000 (DHSS, 1986). The majority of these drugs would be benzodiazepine compounds. If, as a conservative estimate, one quarter of these prescriptions were for long-term users similar to those identified in this sample, then, at a success rate of one in four, the drugs saving could be around £160,000. In England as a whole, this saving could be nearly £3 million in one year. Against this must be set the doctor's time to write the letter or conduct the interview and postage and secretarial costs. However, these costs need not exceed the repeating costs of issuing the prescriptions over several years. The drugs saving would continue as long as no further patients were put onto long-term use.

3. FUTURE WORK

3.1 The use of bibliotherapy

Having established in two published studies (Cormack and Sinnott, 1983; Hopkins et al, 1982) and in the present study that a brief interview or letter from a doctor can be effective in reducing or stopping long-term benzodiazepine use, it would be worthwhile investigating ways of improving the effectiveness of the intervention. Strategies employed by patients for reduction of medication were found to be vague and unsophisticated. Patients who attended group therapy reported specific benefit from the taught strategies and thus there could be advantage in presenting patients with literature about possible alternatives to the use of benzodiazepines.

The leaflet which was given to group members and to patients who requested information at interview with the psychologist could form the basis for a package of information serving the purpose of bibliotherapy. Additional information could be provided either through the post or in interview with the GP at intervals after the initial request. The further communication could serve to maintain the patient's enthusiasm to continue reducing medication and to provide information pertinent to the later stages of reduction.

The kinds of information to be given could include:
    a) information about the drugs and their effects;
    b) how to cut down gradually from the original dose;
    c) how to recognise withdrawal symptoms and how to deal with them;
    d) strategies to employ to induce relaxation.

In home based treatment programmes for agoraphobia, good success, maintained at follow up, has been demonstrated using bibliotherapy (Jannoun et al, 1980). A comparative study of various behavioural treatments for agoraphobia showed the superiority of an approach using minimal professional help, teaching the patient and spouse to deal with the agoraphobic problem with the aid of simple literature (Munby and Johnston, 1980). Thus approaches which give control of the problem to the patient appear to be more effective than those where the therapist determines treatment.

3.2 Expansion of inclusion criteria

In the present study, patients aged over 65 years were excluded because previous work (Cormack, 1981) had found that the older age group responded less well to intervention. However, Giblin and Clift (1983) demonstrated success in helping the over 70's to sleep without hypnotics, through training in relaxation and cognitive approaches. Given these findings, there is no reason to suppose that the older age group should be excluded from future research.

Patients with a known alcohol problem had been excluded from the study because of the concern that alcohol would be substituted for the benzodiazepines. Future work could include an interview from the GP about the potential danger of increasing alcohol use and the current dangers of mixing alcohol and benzodiazepines in terms of psychomotor impairment (Linnoila (1983) demonstrated the enhancement of alcohol effects by benzodiazepines in tests of driving ability). A modification of the doctor's interview could be aimed at general reduction of psychotropic drug intake, starting with either alcohol or benzodiazepines, according to the information gathered at the interview. As alcohol is potentially more hazardous to health, and as the benzodiazepines may have been prescribed to counter some of the effects of the alcohol, alcohol may be the first drug to reduce in most cases.

The minimum time on benzodiazepines was set as one year in this study. It has been shown that tolerance and dependence can develop within a few weeks of normal therapeutic dose (Committee on the Review of Medicines, 1980), therefore, it may be suggested that long-term use could be defined as six months. The average duration of use of benzodiazepines was 12 years, with only five people having a duration of use less than five

years. An investigation of people who had taken the drugs for six months
to two years would be valuable in assessing the prevention of further
long-term use.

3.3 Psychology contribution

Future work by psychologists in the field of long-term benzodiazepine use
should perhaps be directed in other ways. It is important that work on
long-term use should look not only at reducing medication after some
years, but also at preventing the initial prescription. Working with
doctors to enhance their consultation skills and to highlight alternatives
to benzodiazepines that may be attempted by the GP (see Cormack and
Forrest, 1985) could prevent prescribing.

Another avenue of work for psychologists could be in education of the
public about realistic expectations of how life should be. There has
arisen a belief in society that psychological distress should be avoided
at all costs and a view that anxiety is unacceptable (Marinker, 1973).
Pharmaceutical companies have helped to confirm this belief among doctors
through their advertising (Cooperstock, 1987). Perhaps it is now the turn
of psychologists to engage in preventative work through community
education about the role of anxiety in normal behaviour.

REFERENCES

ADAM, K. & OSWALD, I. (1982). A comparison of the effects of clormezanone and nitrazepam on sleep. British Journal of Clinical Pharmacology, 14: 57-65.

ALLGULANDER, C. (1978). Dependence on sedative and hypnotic drugs - a comparative clinical and social study. Acta Psychiatrica Scandinavica, 270 (Supplement): 1-102.

ANDERSON, J.E. (1981). Prescribing of tranquillisers to women and men. Canadian Medical Association Journal, 125: 1229-1232.

ANDERSON, S. & HASLER, J.C. (1979). Counselling in general practice. Journal of the Royal College of General Practitioners, 29: 352-356.

ASHTON, H. (1984). Benzodiazepine withdrawal: an unfinished story. British Medical Journal, 288: 1135-1140. 6ld 5r

AYD, F.J. (1979). Benzodiazepine dependence and withdrawal. Journal of the American Medical Association, 242: 1401-1402.

BALINT, M., HUNT, J., JOYCE, D., MARINKER, M. & WOODCOCK, J. (1970). Treatment or diagnosis. London: Tavistock.

BALTER, M.B., LEVINE, J., & MANHEIMER, F.D. (1974). Cross national study of the extent of anti-anxiety/sedative drug use. New England Journal of Medicine, 290: 769-774.

BASS, M.J. & BASKERVILLE, J.C. (1981). Prescribing of minor tranquillisers for emotional problems in a family practice. Canadian Medical Association Journal, 125: 1225-1226.

BERKELEY, J.S., & RICHARDSON, I.M. (1973). Drug usage in general practice. Journal of the Royal College of General Practitioners, 23: 155-161.

BRADLEY, N.C.A. (1981). Expectations and experience of people who consult in a training practice. Journal of the Royal College of General Practitioners, 31: 420-425.

BREIMER, D.D. (1979). Pharmacokinetics and metabolism of various benzodiazepines used as hypnotics. British Journal of Clinical Pharmacology, 8 (Supplement): 7s-13s.

BREIMER, D.D., BRACHT, H. & DE BOER, A.G. (1977). Plasma level profile of nitrazepam (Mogadon) following oral administration. British Journal of Clinical Pharmacology, 4: 709-711.

CASSANO, G.B. & CONTI, L. (1981). Some considerations on the role of benzodiazepines in the treatment of depression. British Journal of Clinical Pharmacology, 11 (Supplement): 23s-29s.

CATALAN, J., GATH, D., EDMONDS, G. & ENNIS, J. (1984). The effects of non-prescribing of anxiolytics in general practice. 1. Controlled evaluation of psychiatric and social outcome. British Journal of Psychiatry, 144: 593-602.

CATALAN, J. & GATH, D.H. (1985). Benzodiazepines in general practice: time for a decision. British Medical Journal, 290: 1374-1376.

CLARE, A.W. & LADER, M. (Eds) (1982). Psychiatry and general practice. London: Academic Press.

CLARE, A. & WILLIAMS, P. (1981). Factors leading to psychotropic drug prescription. In R. Murray and H. Ghodse (Eds.) The misuse of psychotropic drugs. London: Gaskell, The Royal College of Psychiatrists.

CLIFT, A.D. (1972). Factors leading to dependence on hypnotic drugs. British Medical Journal, 3: 614-617.

COMMITTEE ON THE REVIEW OF MEDICINES (1980). Systematic review of the benzodiazepines. British Medical Journal, 280: 910-912.

COOK, D.G., CUMMINS, R.O., BARTLEY, M.J., et al. (1982). Health of unemployed middle aged men in Great Britain. The Lancet, 5 June, 1290-1294.

COOPERSTOCK, R. (1971). Sex differences in the use of mood modifying drugs: an explanatory model. Journal of Health and Social Behaviour, 12: 238-244.

COOPERSTOCK, R. (1978). Sex differences in psychotropic drug use. Social Science and Medicine, 12B: 179-186.

COOPERSTOCK, R. (1979). Some factors involved in the increased prescribing of psychotropic drugs. In P. Williams and A. Clare (Eds.) Psychosocial disorders in general practice, pp. 161-174. London: Academic Press.

CORMACK, M.A. (1981a). Psychological alternatives to benzodiazepines. Paper presented to the Annual Conference of the Mersyside and North Wales Faculty of the Royal College of General Practitioners. December.

CORMACK, M.A. (1981b). Psychological alternatives to long-term benzodiazepine use. Unpublished Master of Psychology (clinical specialization) thesis, University of Liverpool.

CORMACK, M.A. & SINNOTT, A. (1983). Psychological alternatives to long-term benzodiazepine use. Journal of the Royal College of General Practitioners, 33: 279-281.

CORMACK, M.A. & FORREST, M. (1985). The working relationship between general practitioners and the clinical psychologist. The British Psychological Society Division of Clinical Psychology Newsletter, 48: 33-36.

COSTA, E. (Ed.) (1983). The benzodiazepines. From molecular biology to clinical practice. New York: Raven Press.

CUMMINS, R.O., COOK, D.G., HUME, R.C., & SHAPER, A.G. (1982). Tranquillizer use in middle-aged British men. Journal of the Royal College of General Practitioners, 32: 745-752.

DEADMAN, J. (1984). Factors associated with duration of benzodiazepine use in general practice patients. Unpublished Master of Clinical Psychology thesis, University of Liverpool.

DE BARD, M.L. (1979). Diazepam withdrawal syndrome: a case with psychosis, seizure and coma. American Journal of Psychiatry, 136: 104-105.

DENNIS, P.J. (1979). Monitoring of psychotropic drug prescriptions in general practice. British Medical Journal, 2: 1115-1116.

DHSS. (1986). Health and social services statistics for England. Family Practitioner committee services. London, HMSO.

DUNNELL, K. (1973). Medicine takers and hoarders. Journal of the Royal College of General Practitioners, 23 (Supplement 2: The medical use of psychotropic drugs): 2-9.

EDWARDS, G., CANTOPHER, T. & OLIVIERI, S. (1984). Dependence on psychotropic drugs: an overview. Postgraduate Medical Journal, 60 (Supplement 2): 29-40.

EVANS, J.G. & JARVIS, E.H. (1972). Nitrazepam and the elderly. British Medical Journal, 4: p 487.

FELDMAN, P.E. (1962). An analysis of the efficacy of diazepam. Journal of Neuropsychiatry, 3 (Supplement 1): s62-s67.

FLEMING, D.M & CROSS, K.W. (1984). Psychotropic drug prescribing. Journal of the Royal College of General Practitioners, 34: 216-220.

FREEMAN, G.K. & BUTTON, E.J. (1984). The clinical psychologist in general practice: a six year study of consulting patterns for psychosocial problems. Journal of the Royal College of General Practitioners, 34: 377-380.

GARATTINI, S., MUSSINI, E., MARCUCCI, F., & GUAITANI, A. (1973). Metabolic studies on benzodiazepines in various animal species. In S. Garattini, E. Mussini, L.O. Randall (Eds.) The benzodiazepines. pp 75-97. New York: Raven Press.

GARATTINI, S., MUSSINI, E. & RANDALL, L.O. (1973). The benzodiazepines. New York: Raven Press.

GIBLIN, M.J & CLIFT, A.D. (1983). Sleep without drugs. Journal of the Royal College of General Practitioners, 33: 628-633.

GRAY, J.A. (1979). Anxiety and the brain: not by neurochemistry alone. Psychological Medicine, 9: 605-609.

GRAY, J.A., HOLT, L. & McNAUGHTON, N. (1983). Clinical implications of the experimental pharmacology of the benzodiazepines. In E. Costa (Ed.) The benzodiazepines. From molecular biology to clinical practice. New York: Raven Press.

GREENBLATT, D.J. & SHADER, R.I. (1974). Benzodiazepines in clinical practice. New York: Raven Press. 1974

GREENBLATT, D.J., SHADER, R.I., DIVOLL, M. & HARMATZ, J.S. (1981). Benzodiazepines: a summary of pharmacokinetic properties. British Journal of Clinical Pharmacology, 11 (Supplement) : 11s-16s.

GRIFFITHS, R.R. & ATOR, N.A. (1980). Benzodiazepine self-administration in animals and humans: a comprehensive literature review. United States National Institute on Drug Abuse Research Monographs Series, 33: 22-36.

HAEFELY, W.E. (1980). Biological basis of the therapeutic effects of benzodiazepines. In R.G Priest Benzodiazepines today and tomorrow. pp. 19-45. Lancaster: MTP Press.

HALL, R.C.W. & JOFFE, J.R. (1972). Aberrant response to diazepam: a new syndrome. American Journal of Psychiatry, 129: 738-742.

HALL, R.C.W. & ZISOOK, S. (1981). Paradoxical reactions to benzodiazepines. British Journal of Clinical Pharmacology, 11 (Supplement): 99s-104s.

HARRIS, G., LATHAM, J., McGUINNESS, B. & CRISP, A.H. (1977). The relationship between psychoneurotic status and psychoactive drug prescription in general practice. Journal of the Royal College of General Practitioners, 27: 173-177.

HELMAN, C.G. (1981). Patients' perceptions of psychotropic drugs. Journal of the Royal College of General Practitioners, 31: 107-112.

HEMMINKI, E. (1975). Review of the literature on the factors affecting drug prescribing. Social Science and Medicine, 9: 111-115.

HENDLER, N., CIMINI, C., LONG, T. & LONG, D. (1980). A comparison of cognitive impairment due to benzodiazepines and narcotics. American Journal of Psychiatry, 137: 828-830.

HIGGITT, A., GOLOMBOK, S., FONAGY, P. & LADER, M. (1987). Group treatment of benzodiazepine dependence. British Journal of Addiction, 82: 517-532.

HIGGITT, A.C., LADER, M.H. & FONAGY, P. (1985). Clinical management of benzodiazepine dependence. British Medical Journal, 291: 688-690.

HINDMARCH, I. (1979a). Effects of hypnotic and sleep inducing drugs on objective assessments of human psychomotor performance and subjective appraisals of sleep and early morning behaviour. British Journal of Clinical Pharmacology, 8 (Supplement): 43s-46s.

HINDMARCH, I. (1979b). Some aspects of the effects of clobazam on human psychomotor performance. British Journal of Clinical Pharmacology, 7 (Supplement): 77s-82s.

HINDMARCH, I. (1979c). Benzodiazepines and traffic accidents. British Medical Journal, 2(6191): 671.

HINDMARCH, I. (1981). Psychotropic drugs and psychomotor performance. In R. Murray and H. Ghodse (Eds.) The misuse of psychotropic drugs. London: Gaskell, The Royal College of Psychiatrists.

HINDMARCH, I. (1985). Benzodiazepines: what is missing from the white list? The Pharmaceutical Journal, 234: 506-507.

HINDMARCH, I. & PARROTT, A.C. (1979). The effects of repeated nocturnal doses of clobazam, dipotassium chlorazepate and placebo on subjective ratings of sleep and early morning behaviour and objective measures of arousal, psychomotor performance and anxiety. British Journal of Clinical Pharmacology, 8: 325-329.

HOLLISTER, L.E. (1973). Antianxiety drugs in clinical practice. In S. Garattini et al (Eds.) The benzodiazepines. pp 367-377. New York: Raven Press.

HOLLISTER, L.E. (1981). Benzodiazepines: an overview. British Journal of Clinical Pharmacology, 11 (Supplement 1): 117s-119s.

HOPKINS, D.R., SETHI, K.B.S. & MUCKLOW, J.C. (1982). Benzodiazepine withdrawal in general practice. Journal of the Royal College of General Practitioners, 32: 758-762.

HOWE, J.G. (1980). Lorazepam withdrawal seizures. British Medical Journal, 280: 1163-1164.

INGHAM, J. (1981). Defining the problem. In A. Clare & M. Lader (Eds). Psychiatry and General Practice. London: Academic Press.

IVERSON, L.L. (1983). Biochemical characterization of benzodiazepine receptors. In M.R. Trimble, (Ed.) Benzodiazepines divided. pp 79-85. New York: John Wiley.

IVES, G. (1979). Psychological treatment in general practice. Journal of the Royal College of General Practitioners, 29: 343-351.

JANNOUN, L., MUNBY, M., CATALAN, J. & GELDER, M. (1980). A home based treatment programme for agoraphobia: replication and controlled evaluation. Behaviour Therapy, 11, 294-305.

JOHNSON, D.A.W. (1983). Benzodiazepines in depression. In M.R. Trimble (Ed.) Benzodiazepines divided. New York: John Wiley.

JOHNSON, J. & CLIFT, A.D. (1968). Dependence on hypnotic drugs in general practice. British Medical Journal, 4: 613-617.

JOHNSTONE, E.C., CUNNINGHAM OWENS, D.G., FRITH, C.D., McPHERSON, K., DOWIE, C., RILEY, G. & GOLD, A. (1980). Neurotic illness and its response to anxiolytic and antidepressant treatment. Psychological Medicine, 10: 321-328.

JONES, D.R. (1979). Drugs and prescribing: what the patient thinks. Journal of the Royal College of General Practitioners, 29: 417-419.

KALES, A. (1980). Benzodiazepine hypnotics: carryover effectiveness, rebound insomnia and performance effects. In S.I. Szara & J.P. Ludford (Eds.) Benzodiazepines: a review of research results. National Institute on Drug Abuse, Research Monograph 33, pp 61-69. Washington DC: DHHS.

KALES, A. & SCHARF, M.B. (1973). Sleep laboratory and clinical studies of the effects of benzodiazepines on sleep: flurazepam, diazepam, chlordiazepoxide and RO5-4200. In S. Garattini et al (Eds.) The benzodiazepines. New York: Raven Press. pp 577-625.

KAPLAN, S.A. (1980). Pharmacokinetics of the benzodiazepines. In R.G. Priest Benzodiazepines today and tomorrow. Lancaster: MTP.

KING, D.J., GRIFFITHS, K., REILLY, P.M. & MERRETT, J.D. (1982). Psychotropic drug use in Northern Ireland 1966-80. Psychological Medicine, 12: 819-833.

KNIGHT, R.K. (1970). A survey of outpatient prescribing. Guy's Hospital Reports, 119: 275-287.

KOCH, H.C.H. (1979). Evaluation of behaviour therapy intervention in general practice. Journal of the Royal College of General Practitioners, 29: 337-340.

LADER, M. (1979). Anxiety reduction and sedation: psychophysiological theory. British Journal of Clinical Pharmacology, 7 (Supplement): 99s-105s.

LADER, M. (1981a). Epidemic in the making: benzodiazepine dependence. In G. Tognoni et al (Eds.) The epidemiological impact of psychotropic drugs. pp 313-323. Amsterdam: Elsevier.

LADER, M. (1981b). Benzodiazepine dependence. In R. Murray & H. Ghodse (Eds.) The misuse of psychotropic drugs. London: Gaskell, The Royal College of Psychiatrists.

LADER, M. (1982). Benzodiazepine dependence. Psychiatry in practice, 1(9).

LADER, M. (1983a). Benzodiazepines, psychological functioning and dementia. In M.R. Trimble (Ed.) Benzodiazepines divided. New York: John Wiley.

LADER, M. (1983b). Long term use and problems of withdrawal. MIMS magazine, 28-31.

LADER, M.H., CURRY, S. & BAKER, W.J. (1980). Physiological and psychological effects of clorazepate in man. British Journal of Clinical Pharmacology, 9: 83-90.

LADER, M.H., RON, M. & PETURSSON, H. (1984). Computed axial brain tomography in long-term benzodiazepine users. Psychological Medicine, 14: 203-206.

LEY, R. (1985). Agoraphobia, the panic attack and the hyperventilation syndrome. Behaviour Research and Therapy, 23(1): 79-81.

LINDSAY, W.R., GAMSU, C.V., McLAUGHLIN, E., HOOD, E.M. & ESPIE, C.A. (1987). A controlled trial of treatment for generalised anxiety. British Journal of Clinical Psychology, 26, 3-15.

LINNOILA, M. (1983). Benzodiazepines and performance. In E. Costa (Ed.) The benzodiazepines. From molecular biology to clinical practice. New York: Raven Press.

LYNCH, M.A., LINDSAY, J. & OUNSTED, C. (1975). Tranquillisers causing aggression. British Medical Journal, 1: 266.

MADDEN, J.S. (1979). A guide to alcohol and drug dependence. Bristol: John Wright and Sons.

MALPAS, A., ROWAN, A.J., JOYCE, C.R.B. & SCOTT, D.F. (1970). Persistent behavioural and electrocephalographic changes after single doses of nitrazepam and amylobarbitone sodium. British Medical Journal, 2: 762-764.

MANASSE, A.P. (1974). Repeat prescriptions in general practice. Journal of the Royal College of General Practitioners, 24: 203-207.

MAPES, E. (Ed.) (1980). Prescribing practice and drug usage. London: Croom Helm.

MAPES, R.E. & WILLIAMS, W.O. (1979). The changing pattern of general practitioner drug prescribing in the NHS in England from 1970-1975. Journal of the Royal College of General Practitioners, 29: 406-412.

MARINKER, M. (1973). The doctor's role in prescribing. In The Royal College of General Practitioners, The medical use of psychotropic drugs. Journal of the Royal College of General Practitioners, 23 (Supplement 2): 26-29.

MARKS, J., & NICHOLSON, A.N. (1984). Drugs and insomnia. British Medical Journal, 288: 261.

MEICHENBAUM, D.M. (1977). Cognitive behaviour medication: an integrative approach. New York: Plenum Press.

MELLINGER, G.D. & BALTER, M.B. (1981). Prevalence and patterns of use of psychotherapeutic drugs: results from a 1979 national survey of American adults. In G. Tognoni et al (Eds.) The epidemiological impact of psychotropic drugs. Amsterdam: Elsevier. pp 117-135.

MELVILLE, A. (1980). Reducing whose anxiety? A study of the relationship between repeat prescribing of minor tranquillisers and doctors' attitudes. In E. Mapes (Ed.) Prescribing practice and drug usage. London: Croom Helm.

MENDELSON, W.B. (1980). The use and misuse of sleeping pills. New York: Plenum.

MORGAN, K. & OSWALD, I. (1982). Anxiety caused by a short-life hypnotic. British Medical Journal, 284 (6320): 942.

MUNBY, M. & JOHNSTON, D.W. (1980). Agoraphobia: the long term follow up of behavioural treatment. British Journal of Psychiatry, 137. 418-427.

MURDOCH, J.C. (1980). The epidemiology of prescribing in an urban general practice. Journal of the Royal College of General Practitioners, 30: 593-602.

MURRAY, J., WILLIAMS, P. & CLARE, A. (1982). Health and social characteristics of long-term psychotropic drug takers. Social Science and Medicine, 16(18): 1595-1598.

MURRAY, R., GHODSE, H. et al (Eds.) (1981). The misuse of psychotropic drugs. London: Gaskell, The Royal College of Psychiatrists.

McALLISTER, T.A. & PHILIP, A.E. (1975). The clinical psychologist in a health centre: one year's work. British Medical Journal, 4: 513-514.

NICHOLSON, A.N. (1979a). Hypnotics today. Practitioner, 223: 479-484.

NICHOLSON, A.N. (1979b). Performance studies with diazepam and its hydroxylated metabolites. British Journal of Clinical Pharmacology, 8 (Supplement) : 39s-42s.

NICHOLSON, A.N. (1981). The use of short- and long-acting hypnotics in clinical medicine. British Journal of Clinical Pharmacology, 11 (Supplement 1): 61s-69s.

NICHOLSON, A.N. & SPENCER, M.B. (1982). Psychological impairment and low dose benzodiazepine treatment. British Medical Journal, 285: 99.

OSWALD, I. (1983). Benzodiazepines and sleep. In M.R. Trimble (Ed.) Benzodiazepines divived. New York: John Wiley. pp 261-276.

OWEN, R.T. & TYRER, P. (1983). Benzodiazepine dependence: a review of the evidence. Drugs, 25: 385-398.

PARISH, P.A. (1973). What influences have led to increased prescribing of psychotropic drugs? Journal of the Royal College of General Practitioners, 23 (Supplement 2) 49-57.

PARISH, P.A. (1981). The use of psychotropic drugs in general practice. In A. W. Clare & M. Lader (Eds.) Psychiatry and General Practice. London: Academic Press.

PETURSSON, H. & LADER, M. (1981). Withdrawal from long term benzodiazepine treatment. British Medical Journal, 283: 643-645.

PETURSSON, H. & LADER, M. (1984). Dependence on tranquillizers. _Maudsley_
Monographs 28. Oxford: Oxford University Press.

PRESCOTT, L.F. (1983). Safety of the benzodiazepines. In E. Costa (Ed.)
The benzodiazepines. From molecular biology to clinical practice.
New York: Raven Press.

PRIEST, R.G. (1980). _Benzodiazepines today and tomorrow_. Lancaster: MTP
press.

PURPURA, R.P. (1981). Approaches in the evaluation of hypnotics: studies
with triazolam. _British Journal of Clinical Pharmacology_, _11_
(Supplement): 37s-42s.

RAPEE, R.M. (1985). A case of panic disorder treated with breathing
retraining. _Journal of Behaviour Therapy and Experimental_
Psychiatry, _16_(1): 63-65.

RAPOPORT, J. (1979). Patients' expectations and intentions to
self-medicate. _Journal of the Royal College of General_
Practitioners, _29_: 468-472.

RICKELS, K. (1973). Predictors of response to benzodiazepines in anxious
outpatients. In S. Garattini et al (Eds.) _The benzodiazepines_. New
York: Raven Press.

RICKELS, K. (1980). Benzodiazepines: clinical use patterns. In S. Szara
& J.P. Ludford (Eds.) _Benzodiazepines: a review of research results_.
National Institute on Drug Abuse. Research Monograph 33, Washington
DC. DHHS.

RICKELS, K. (1981). Are benzodiazepines overused and abused? _British_
Journal of Clinical Pharmacology, _11_ (Supplement) : 71s-83s.

RICKELS, K. (1980). Benzodiazepines in the treatment of anxiety: North
American experiences. In E. Costa (Ed.) _The benzodiazepines. From_
molecular biology to clinical practice. New York: Raven Press.

ROBSON, M.H., FRANCE, R. & BLAND, M. (1984). Clinical psychologist in
primary care: controlled clinical and economic evaluation. _British_
Medical Journal, _288_: 1805-1808.

ROTH, T., ZORICK, F., SICKLESTEEL, J. & STEPANSKI, E.(1981). Effects of
benzodiazepines on sleep and wakefulness. _British Journal of_
Clinical Pharmacology, _11_ (Supplement) : 31s-35s.

ROTHSTEIN, E., COBBLE, J.C. & SAMPSON, N. (1976). Chlordiazepoxide: long
term use in alcoholism. _Annals of the New York Academy of Science_,
_273_: 381-384.

SALKIND, M.R. (1981). Anxiety in the community. In R. Murray & H. Ghodse
(Eds.) _The misuse of psychotropic drugs_. London: Gaskell, The Royal
College of Psychiatrists.

SALKIND, M.R., HANKS, G.W. & SILVERSTONE, J.T. (1979). Evaluation of the
effects of clobazam, a 1,5 benzodiazepine, on mood and psychomotor
performance in clinically anxious patients in general practice.
British Journal of Clinical Pharmacology, _7_ (Supplement): 113s-118s.

SHADER, R.I. & GREENBLATT, D.J. (1981). The use of benzodiazepines in
clinical practice. _British Journal of Clinical Pharmacology_, _11_
(Supplement 1): 5s-9s.

SHEPHERD, M., COOPER, B., BROWN, A.C. & KALTON, G. (1966). Psychiatric illness in general practice. London: Oxford University Press.

SHEPHERD, M., HARWIN, B.G., DEPLA, C. & CAIRNS, V. (1979). Social work and the primary care of mental disorder. Psychological Medicine, 9: 661-669.

SKEGG, D.C.G., DOLL, R. & PERRY, J. (1977). Use of medicines in general practice. British Medical Journal, 1: 1561.

SKEGG, D.C.G., RICHARDS, S.M. & DOLL, R. (1979). Minor tranquillisers and road accidents. British Medical Journal, 1: 917-919.

STIMSON, G.V. (1976). Doctor-patient interaction and some problems for prescribing. Journal of the Royal College of General Practitioners, 26 (Supplement 1): 88-96.

SWIFT, C.G. (1981). Psychotropic drugs and the elderly. In G. Tognoni et al (Eds.) The epidemiological impact of psychotropic drugs. Amsterdam: Elsevier.

SZARA, S.I. & LUDFORD, J.P. (Eds.). (1980). Benzodiazepines: a review of research results. National Institute on Drug Abuse, Research Monograph 33, Washington DC: DHHS.

TEARE SKINNER, P. (1984). Skills not pills: learning to cope with anxiety symptoms. Journal of the Royal College of General Practitioners, 34: 258-260.

TEDESCHI, G., GRIFFITHS, A.N., SMITH, A.T. & RICHENS, A. (1985). The effect of repeated doses of temazepam and nitrazepam on human psychomotor performance. British Journal of Clinical Pharmacology, 20: 361-367.

TESSLER, R., STOKES, R. & PIETRAS, M. (1978). Consumer response to Valium. Drug Therapy, 8: 178-183.

THOMPSON, D.J. (1985). Comparison of drug treatment (clobazam) and relaxation therapy in the management of anxiety. Preliminary communication. Royal Society of Medicine International Congress and Symposium Series, 74: 101-104.

TOGNONI, G., BELLANTUONO, C. & LADER, M. (Eds.) (1981). The epidemiological impact of psychotropic drugs. Amsterdam: Elsevier.

TRETHOWAN, W.H. (1977). The role of the psychologist in the Health Service. HMSO, London.

TRIMBLE, M.R. (Ed.) (1983). Benzodiazepines divided. New York: John Wiley.

TYRER, P. (1978). Drug treatment of psychiatric patients in general practice. British Medical Journal, 2: 1008-1010.

TYRER, P.J. (1984). Benzodiazepines on trial. British Medical Journal, 288: 1101-1102.

TYRER, P., RUTHERFORD, D. & HUGGETT, T. (1981). Benzodiazepine withdrawal symptoms and propranolol. Lancet, i(8219): 520-522.

TYRER, P., OWEN, R. & DAWLING, S. (1983). Gradual withdrawal of diazepam after long-term therapy. Lancet, i: 1402-1406.

TYRER, P. & SEIVEWRIGHT, N. (1984). Identification and management of benzodiazepine dependence. Postgraduate Medical Journal, 60 (Supplement 2): 41-46.

VARNAM, M. (1981). Psychotropic prescribing. What am I doing? Journal of the Royal College of General Practitioners, 31: 480-483.

WAYDENFELD, D. & WAYDENFELD, S.W. (1980). Counselling in general practice. Journal of the Royal College of General Practitioners, 30: 671-677.

WILLIAMS, P. (1978). Physical ill health and psychotropic drug prescription - a review. Psychological Medicine, 8: 683-693.

WILLIAMS, P. (1980). Recent trends in the prescribing of psychotropic drugs. Health Trends, 12: 6-7.

WILLIAMS, P. (1981). Trends in the prescribing of psychotropic drugs. In R. Murray, H. Ghodse et al (Eds.) The misuse of psychotropic drugs. London: Gaskell, The Royal College of Psychiatrists.

WILLIAMS, P. (1983). Factors influencing the duration of treatment with psychotropic drugs in general practice: a survival analysis approach. Psychological Medicine, 13: 623-633.

WILLIAMS, P. & CLARE, A. (Eds.) (1979). Psychosocial disorders in general practice. London: Academic Press.

WILLIAMS, P., MURRAY, J. & CLARE, A. (1982). A longitudinal study of psychotropic drug prescription. Psychological Medicine, 12: 201-206.

WINOKUR, A., RICKELS, K., GREENBLATT, D.J., SNYDER, P.J. & SCHATZ, N.J. (1980). Withdrawal reaction from long-term, low-dosage administration of diazepam. Archives of General Psychiatry, 37: 101-105.

WITTENBORN, J.R. (1979). Effects of benzodiazepines on psychomotor performance. British Journal of Clinical Pharmacology, 7 (Supplement): 61s-67s.

WORLD HEALTH ORGANISATION. (1974). Expert committee on drug dependence. Twentieth report. WHO technical report series Number 551. Geneva: WHO.

APPENDIX

Reasons subjects gave for taking tablets

Initial	Maintaining
1. very nervy	*
2. lousy sleeper	to help sleeping
3. husband died	looked after ailing mother
4. got all panicky	worry (compulsive eater)
5. periods of bad sleep	difficulty in sleeping
6. agoraphobia	agoraphobia
7. afraid, poor sleeper, nerves	insomnia, husband had heart attack
8. mother died, alcoholic husband	alcoholic husband, spinal problem (pain)
9. nervous wreck	fear, panic, loneliness
10. depressed and anxious	panics in crowds, bored, depressed, work stresses
11. agoraphobia	tension in stomach
12. coping with demented mother	nervy, reliant on pills
13. agoraphobia	placebo effect
14. nervous breakdown	worry, panic, depression, two broken marriages, invalid mother
15. husband died	worries, placebo effect
16. could not sleep after car accident	pain in stomach
17. prescribed Ativan in hospital then sister died	clung to them
18. agoraphobia	lonely, frightened, could not sleep
19. nursing sick relatives	heart attack, stress, anxious
20. felt could not swallow and panic	habit
21. mother died	fear of fear ("what if ...")
22. cervical spondylosis – muscular spasms	pain and muscular spasms
23. baby died	got into habit of taking them

24. new medication for heart problem   panic attacks, agoraphobia

25. thought of people dying   thought of people dying

26. nerves, helped to sleep   help to sleep, probably psychological

27. migraine   get worked up (tense)

28. depressed   take them to get to sleep

29. depressed, anxious, etc.   feels washed out, anxious, etc.

30. high blood pressure, middle ear infection   doctor said to continue

31. could not cope after daughter born   panics in shops

32. nervous after car accident   worry, caring for ageing mother

33. *   nervous in the day

34. could not sleep, headaches, daughter pestered at school   problems with daughter, feeling depressed

35. panicked, not normally like that   *

36. operation then husband died   lacking energy

37. post natal depression   nerves

38. in hospital after car accident   could be psychological

39. father died   anxious

40. brother died   family upsets, agoraphobia, another brother died

* - no reason given